STANDING TALL ABOVE DRUGS

A MODERN CRUSADE

☙☙☙☙☙☙☙☙☙☙☙☙☙☙☙☙☙☙☙☙

Robert T. Wall

COLUMBIA COLLEGE LIBRARY

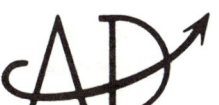

ACCELERATED DEVELOPMENT INC.
Publishers
Muncie   Indiana

STANDING TALL ABOVE DRUGS
A MODERN CRUSADE

© Copyright 1989 by Accelerated Development Inc.

1 2 3 4 5 6 7 8 9 10

Printed in the United States of America

All rights reserved. No part of this book may be reproduced or transmitted by any form or means, electronic or mechanical, including photocopying, recording, or by an informational storage and retrieval system, without permission in writing from Accelerated Development Inc.

Technical Development: Tanya Dalton
                                 Sandra Gilmore
                                 Delores Kellogg
                                 Marguerite Mader
                                 Sheila Sheward

Library of Congress Cataloging in Publication Data

      Wall, Robert T., 1931-
         Standing tall above drugs.

         Includes index.
         1. Drug abuse—United States—Prevention. 2. Self-actualization (Psychology) 3. Health. 4. Life style. I. title.
      HV5825.W38126 1988   613.8'3   88-70587
      ISBN 0-915202-82-4

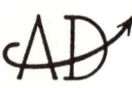

ACCELERATED DEVELOPMENT Inc., PUBLISHERS
3400 Kilgore

TABLE OF CONTENTS

PART I   ALPHA . . . THE BEGINNING 1

1   RISING ABOVE THE CROWD 3
    An Introduction to the Addiction Dilemma 4
    Still More Statistical Evidence 6
    What Is It Costing Us? 8
    Stick 'Em Up, Brother! 9
    Three Legs of the Problem 10
    Like the Beat, The Search for Excellence Goes On 12
    Paradox of Adolescence 14
    And Yet Another County Heard From 15
    Some Medical Evidence 16
    The Economics of It 17
    Too Many Cooks in the Kitchen? 21
    Any Progress in Sight? 23
    Focus on Prevention 24
    A Friend in Need 25
    United We Stand 26
    To Thine Own Self Be True 27
    One for All, All for One 29
    A Crusade Looking for Crusaders 30
    The Crusader System—21st Century Style 32
    Summary 34

2   NO IS NOT ENOUGH 35
    More Than Blood Out of a Turnip 36
    A Case History 36
    Getting On With Balancing 38

What is a Crusader? 39
Sometimes, Mother Knows Best 40
In God We Trust 42
There, But for the Grace of God 44
From a Teacher's Point of View 45
Put a Little Love in Your Life 46
We've Got Your Number 49
Two Heads Are Better Than One 50
The World of Work Offers Employee Assistance 53
Connecting Personal Issues to Corporate
 and National Interests 55
From the Hallowed Halls of Corporate American 56
On a More Personal Level 57
A Gift to Be Nurtured 59
Summary 61

3 CHECK UNDER THE HOOD, PLEASE 63

The Inner Motivation: Basic Values 64
The Nature of Motivation 65
The Interconnection of Learning and Change 69
One Man's Meat 70
Home is What You Make It 74
Creativity as a Discipline 79
How People Use Their Influence 81
Another Place, Another View of Influence 81
Adults as Learners and Teachers 83
When All Else Fails 85
Men Against Women—One More Time 86
Keep Those Cards and Letter Coming 87
Reaching a State of Balance 89
Music to Your Ears 90
Summary 92

4 LIVING ON THE EDGE ... 93

- The Treatment of the Thrill Reality ... 96
- The Other Side of the Coin ... 97
- Another Time, Another Setting ... 98
- On the Personal Side of It ... 99
- A Poet in Our Midst ... 101
- Snapshot ... 102
- The Next Steps ... 103
- Parents Look Back and Wonder—What If... ... 104
- The Path to Power is Strewn with Bodies ... 104
- Viva Le Difference ... 105
- The Alpha Stages—Awareness and Options ... 106
- Another Crusader in Disguise ... 108
- Pulling Back the Covers on Insidious Relationships ... 109
- The Alpha Process—A Starting Place ... 111
- Decisions, Decisions, Decisions ... 113
- Summary ... 115

PART II BECKONING ... GROWTH OPTIONS ... 117

5 THE KINDRED SPIRIT ... 119

- What's Really Good for Each Family Member? ... 122
- The Connecting of These Loose Ends is Synergy ... 124
- A Young Shoot Grows into a Willow Plant ... 124
- What Does Erik Erickson Say About Prevention? ... 128
- Guidelines are Necessary to Practicing Good Values ... 131
- A Game Plan for New Parents ... 133
- Different Types of Families ... 134
  - Family Number One ... 134
  - Family Number Two ... 135
  - Family Number Three ... 135
  - Family Number Four ... 135
  - Family Number Five ... 135
  - Family Number Six ... 136
  - Family Number Seven ... 136

The Caring Family	136
Giving Up the Responsibility	138
Neoteny as a Model for Family Growth	140
The 2/4/2 Game	142
What is Neoteny?	144
Summary	144

6 SESAME STREET REVISITED ... 145

Television as a Teacher	146
Turning Negatives into Positives	147
The Art of Inclusion	152
Accessing Energy	154
Inner Struggles	155
Self Indulgence	155
Incessant Talking	156
Reacting to Pressure	156
Game Playing	157
Victim Association	157
The Wisdom and Serenity Model	158
Wisdom	159
Serenity	160
Blunderers, Madmen, and Other Feeble Attempts	161
Summary	162

7 SIGNS OF THE TIMES ... 163

Need for Conflict Resolution Skills	164
Teaching and Law Enforcement: Companions?	166
New Ways of Managing Conflict	168
The Power of Concentration	171
Stress and Concentration Relationship	172
Time Waits for No One	174
How We Structure Time	175
Best Use of Time	179
Summary	180

8 GETTING TO THE HEART OF THE MATTER 181

External Threat 182
Collision of Two Worlds 182
Status of Escalating Health Care Costs 183
The 120-Year-Old Man 185
Survey of the New Age Generation 186
Finding and Measuring the Missing Link 191
Fix Only What's Broken 192
The Safety Net 193
When Are We Going to Learn? 194
The Helpful Computer 195
A Management Lesson 197
Holding Out the Promise 198
Shaping the Corporate Lifestyle 199
Changing the Bureaucratic System and Mind 201
Summary 204

PART III COMMITMENT . . . A SYNERGISTIC PATH 205

9 BREAKING INTO THE PERFECT CIRCLE 207

If a Star, The Least You Can Do is Shine 208
Synergy Skills Survey 209
    Scoring 212
Synergy Skills Scoring Interpretations 216
    Interpretations for Self-Image 216
    Interpretation for Professional Style 217
    Interpretation for Syngery Profile 217
        1. *Job/Results Clarity (Related to the need of clarity)* 218
        2. *Work Plans/Schedules (Related to
            the need of achievement)* 219
        3. *Problem Solving (Related to the need of industry)* 220
        4. *Indicators/Standards (Related to the need of integrity)* 221
        5. *Feedback/Evaluation (Related to the need of control)* 222
        6. *Data Analysis (Related to the need of curiosity)* 223
        7. *Data Collection (Related to the need of trust)* 224
        8. *Know Needs of Others (Related to the need of intimacy)* 225
        9. *Close the Process (Related to the need of generativity)* 225
        10. *Knowing Self Needs (Related to the need of self identity)* ... 226
        11. *Keep Process Open (Related to the need of autonomy)* 227
        12. *Risk Taking (Related to the need of initiative)* 228
The Road to Peak Performance 229

Getting to Know Yourself	232
Values Survey and Profile	233
Visiting an Attic	241
Mentoring: A Dutch Uncle	245
Overcoming Negatives	246
Changing the Triggers	247
Combine Your Needs to Create Synergy	251
The Wrong Path	253
A Way of Life for the Sidetracker	254
Summary	258

10 CAPTURE THE MOMENT ... 261

Introducing the Planning Process	262
The Art of Disciplined Participation	264
Investing in Children	266
Hope Rises and Expectations Grow	267
Listening to the Message	269
The Beat of a Different Drummer	270
Can Schools Change?	271
The Spirituality Aspect	273
Summary	273

11 STRETCHING THE PROCESS ... 275

Making Each Move Count	276
Keep Home Fires Burning and Burning	277
The Universal Measurement	278
The Establishment Counts, Too	279
The Visual Aids Are Immediate	282
The Visualization Index	283
Values and Synergy Connection	284
Index for Health and Performance	286
A Nuclear Holocaust?	288
Patriotism Generates Energy	289
Evaluation is a Matter of Feedback	292
Getting Closer, Sooner	295
Summary	296

12 STAR SPANGLED SPIRIT ... 297

- A Crusader's Personal Game Plan ... 298
- A Working Model ... 299
- Establish a Baseline ... 301
- The Next Step is Mental Health ... 305
- Crusading Spirit... Standing Tall in a Crowd ... 306
- Integrating Skills and Motivation ... 307
- Measured Commitment ... 309
- Use Short Time Frames ... 311
- Include Calculated Risk ... 312
- Connect to Other Systems ... 312
- Realizing Your Potential ... 313
    - Rational Skills ... 314
    - Intuitive Skills ... 317
- What's Expected of One Who Stands Tall ... 320
- Celebrate ... 320
- Summary ... 321

INDEX ... 323

ABOUT THE AUTHOR ... 331

LIST OF FIGURES

2.1	Numerology instruction for determining your personal year	52
3.1	Illustration of how energy works through the personality	72
3.2	Rational and intuitive skills and related needs	75
3.3	Illustrated sphere of influence	80
6.1	Stages of relationships	148
7.1	A parent-child discussion model	169
8.1	Graphic description of the values/skills/issues corporate lifestyles model	203
9.1	Synergy Skills Summary	210
9.2	Sample of a completed Synergy Skills Graph	212
9.3	Synergy Skills Graph to be completed	213
9.4	Sample of the Three Thermometer Graphs	214
9.5	Three Thermometer Graphs to be completed	215
9.6	Synergy Profile—a schematic representation of potential indicators as shown by intensity in each of twelve synergy skills	230
9.7	Values Survey instrument	234
9.8	Deborah's Synergy Profile	243
9.9	A personality model	248
9.10	Sphere of Influence Cone	256
10.1	Core Value Profile	269
11.1	Health and Performance Index	286
11.2	Three essentials in synergy—needs, skills and issues	291
11.3	Values Tracking System	295
12.1	Conflict Resolution Model	308

PART I
ALPHA...
THE BEGINNING

CHAPTER 1

RISING ABOVE THE CROWD

The stars were shining brightly in a black sky as Tommy Ward slowly opened his eyes. He caught his breath as the pain hit his mind. **"Must have sprained the ankle,"** he muttered to no one—he was alone in the car. **"Better get this car back on the road,"** again talking aloud.

A voice from outside interrupted his effort to start the car. **"What'ya trying to do?"** the stranger asked. **"Your car's on its side and I'd say it was totalled from the looks of things,"** the newcomer added.

The wail of the police siren broke the silence and its growing insistence gave Tommy a new perception of his dilemma. He was intoxicated, injured, and likely to be arrested for driving under the influence. And yet he was lucky—no one else was injured, insurance would cover most of the damage, and within a few days his parents would forget it and no one would be giving it a second thought.

"I dropped my cigarette," he explained to the officer, **"and when I bent to pick it up I must have missed the curve and rolled it down the embankment."** The sheriff's deputy wrote solemnly on his accident clipboard as the whirling red and yellow lights crossed their faces.

"How much have you had to drink tonight," the deputy asked matter of factly.

"Oh not much...couple a beers over the course of the night," he lied.

"Smoke any dope?" the law man persisted.

The old paranoia jolted Tommy as he suddenly remembered the baggie of marijuana tucked under the front seat. A look into the deputy's steady gaze told Tommy he'd better not carry this too far. *"Yeh, I had a couple of hits at the party, not a whole joint—I don't do much dope,"* continuing his cover-up.

"Mind if I look around," the officer said, waving his flashlight into the car.

Tommy went limp and he put his hand on the car to steady himself. *"Nah, go ahead,"* Tom groaned.

"I can do that later," the deputy said. *"We'd better get you to the hospital and have that leg looked at."*

AN INTRODUCTION TO THE ADDICTION DILEMMA

This story, or one like it involving drugs, alcohol, and cigarettes, is repeated throughout the country about every hour on the average, highlighting the severity of America's addiction dilemma. Not every driver is as lucky as the young person in the opening scenario. Many are killed, maimed permanently and in other ways seriously destroying lives. The statistics on drugs, alcohol, and nicotine speak for themself:

> 40,000 people will die directly from alcohol addiction this and every year;
>
> 43% of all adolescents experiment with beer and wine;
>
> 23% of all adolescents have tried "hard stuff";
>
> 90% of those who drink also smoke cigarettes;

350,000 people are dying each year from smoke-related illnesses; and

smoking causes blood, gastro-intestinal, cancer, respiratory, and cardiac diseases in growing percentages annually

Figures on drug use and abuse are not as high—fewer than a thousand persons will die this year from drug addiction—but the violence and unsavory activity of the problem are taking their toll and more than their share of concern from American politicians and parents. School officials acknowledge the trouble, but they are showing a little less concern because of more immediate problems on their plates such as grade scores, salaries, classroom size, professionalism, understaffing, and other labor/management exigencies. Some teachers get involved, other feign ignorance.

An estimated 1.6 million youngsters in junior high school will put themselves at risk to substance addiction this year. They will experiment with drugs because adolescence is a time of experimentation. Young people want to grow up and that takes the experience of trial and error. Without guidance, care, and consideration, they'll likely wind up as one of a national statistic.

Without argument, America has a serious problem of substance abuse, and relatively little is being done to prevent it. These are the pillars on which the premise rests:

1. substance addiction persists in this country because no coordinated effort exists amongst parents, teachers, and government to combat it within realistic expectations;

2. the major effort by the government to curtail the supply of drugs into this country is expensive, at best, and inefficient, at worst;

3. supply and demand sides of the issue are intertwined and both offer insights into how the dilemma can be resolved; and

4. a system is needed to help adolescents develop the strength of character—a philosophy—to resist the temptation of substances, on one hand, and to capitalize on more productive lifestyle options, on the other.

This simply-stated proposition must be both tough-handed and high-minded. To be both suggests the need for a conclusive understanding of duality—both sides of the issue—a yin yang of it. Only with all arguments on the table can good intentions and actions overcome an insidious evil. Like dragging Dracula into sunlight, the task is formidable. But the energy is there.

A rebirth in national patriotism is evident and a new sense of spirituality wafts across the nation's young parents and teens. **With these energies integrated** into a system, people will focus their attention and will on drug, alcohol, and nicotine abuse. By capturing people's focused energy, the battle can be successfully waged. Without a crusading fervor, however, the problem will wax and wane, undermining the nation's youthful potential. It's this one step forward, one back that is most debilitating.

STILL MORE STATISTICAL EVIDENCE

One fortunate fact of life is that young people eventually grow up and out of the six or seven years of adolescence. On the down side, not all survive. Of the 5,000 teen suicide last year, 76% were drug or alcohol related. While not everyone who drinks or does drugs will become an addict, quite clearly psychoactive drugs are dangerous. Even in families where firm, loving social standards are in place, kids get addicted. Where little or no acceptable norms to understand and follow are present, the risks are increased proportionately. While attempting to halt the flow of illegal drugs into this country, more must be done to develop young people capable of resisting the impulse.

You would have to be a Rip Van Winkle not to understand the devastation that substance abuse causes in this country and all over the world every year. The U.S. had to fight this problem almost single-handedly until very recently when addiction in Europe and Asia became a serious family problem.

Part of the problem is growing up—it's a tough and painful time for kids and parents alike.

Another part is our culture—we've always lived on the edge and seem to enjoy the risks and thrills that go with it. Americans portray the ultimate in pioneering and entrepreneurial spirit. This combination is conducive to baiting the addiction trap.

But just what is addiction? Who can get addicted? Can we get rid of this problem by throwing money at it and leaving it at that? Or is it more complex than we've been led to believe?

First question on addiction: Medical experts say it's a process of becoming so dependent on some substance that the user is unable to physically, intellectually, and emotionally stop using it. Some authorities say some addicts are physically hooked, while others claim that some are emotionally snared. In either case, the important thing to know is that once addicted, to shake the habit is mighty difficult.

Generally, the person who takes to pills, alcohol, or smoking builds a tolerance, then a dependence and in the end is addicted—unable to make the choice of whether or not to use.

Alcoholics Anonymous (AA), which is the leading organization for self-treatment of alcohol addicts, says the disease is incurable. Once you get it, you've got it for life. Narcotics, on the other hand, may or may not be curable. Not enough data is around to make scientific conclusions despite nearly 30 years of research. To compound the issue, there's heroin. Treatment for heroin addiction is also addictive.

Users tell us some addictions are solely physical, while some are physical and emotional. Some drugs are, according to the abusers, easy to "kick" on a physical level, but the addicts can't seem to work out the emotional aspects of their problem. They're making a statement about the emotional side of their make-up, which is a major criterion for the recovery process. More about that later.

Anyway you look at it, addiction is a serious, dangerous, and pervasive problem facing this country with no short-term solution in sight.

WHAT IS IT COSTING US?

The costs of addiction are incalculable. Estimates have such a wide-ranging sweep that it means little to print them. But some of the facts and figures will provide a clue to the monumental size of the economics involved.

Some 15 million Americans (10 million men and 5 million women) suffer from alcoholism, which recently has been labeled an incurable disease like AIDS and herpes. Another 20 million are considered moderate to heavy drinkers—ranging from two to six drinks a day. These same adults are role models for young Americans. There's an abundance of evidence that causally links drinking to marijuana to hard drugs.

What it's doing to teens in America is this: the somewhat suspect goal of getting drunk four or five times a year has risen from 10% in 1960 to 19% in 1975 and 27% in 1986. The critical mass is growing and growing. Educational efforts are keeping a record number away from drinking, yet more than ever start— the wax and wane syndrome.

This tendency in kids to purposefully go out and "hang one on" is lethal because of their fragile state of physical, emotional, and mental development. Whether they are on alcohol or drugs, the ability to think and work through life's problem is subverted at a time when a youngster needs to learn how to problem solve rather than find quick escape from life's seeming endless array of trouble. Again, emotions and feelings rear an ugly head. The emotional aspect of adolescence is what trips up the teen. Without adult coping mechanisms and techniques, the adolescent, puzzled about new-felt emotions, is a prime target for a dealer.

Once addicted, adolescents generally run out of money and resort to a growing habit of crime. It starts with stealing funds from the family and evolves into street crime, including dealing drugs to peers and companions as they build their own feeder network of income to supply their new habit.

STICK 'EM UP, BROTHER!

So they travel from family to the street. Studies by the Baltimore police indicated the lower, smaller, the drug use, the fewer the crimes. Conversely, more use means more crime and more severe crime. Burglaries turn to strong arm robbery to assault with a weapon to violent crimes with intent to kill. Amongst criminals, addicts are six times more likely to commit a crime than non-addicts.

Of the 400,000 persons arrested in 1986 for possession of drugs including marijuana, some 15% were convicted. The cost is $55,000 a year to keep each offender in prison, not counting productivity lost, upkeep of the criminal justice system, treatment, and crime prevention. That's about the same price tag as a four-year college education at prestigious Harvard or Stanford. Have we got our national priorities well ordered?

Because drugs usually result in other problems in school, the drop-out is another economic calamity. Loss of interest, truancy, fights, and other irrational behavior become apparent. A school drop-out not only deprives the nation of a productive future citizen, he or she adds another cost in the welfare arena and becomes a double burden for the taxpayer.

Another feature of the double cost can be seen right on the insurance premium, whether the individual pays or the employer does. High cost patients in hospitals account for 80% of the resources allotted there. They also are generally the smokers. Ills associated with smoking are the high cost ailments. Non-smokers help underwrite the insurance coverage for smokers without a vote on the matter. That's hardly democratic.

When you look at the docket in Family Court, the place where non-felony cases are taken, 45% involve deliquency and fully one-half of the traffic there is linked directly to alcohol and drugs. Most of the time, more than one family member is at fault. That means a parent or a brother or a sister are involved in using and abusing.

THREE LEGS OF THE PROBLEM

No longer does one need to doubt that adolescence, alcohol, drugs and nicotine combine to make a scenario which unfairly and perhaps immorally infringes on personal, family, and societal freedoms. Having said that, an examination of each factor individually will flare more light on the argument. Take adolescence first.

Child development authority Erik Erikson pointed out 45 years ago that each of us grows into adulthood as an unique and particularly individual personality. Erikson went on to describe the patterns or stages of growth that we all follow to become independent grown-ups. Sociologists, psychologists, teachers, counselors, and others who work with adolescents and their families credit Erikson's research with helping them better understand the dynamics of child development.

What Erikson discovered about kids is that each passes through eight specific stages, lasting between two to four years generally, learning a set of skills, which prepares the child for adulthood. For instance, he noted, and others have confirmed time and again, that if a child received an appropriate amount of physical and emotional comfort and stroking from birth, he or she develops a **trusting nature.** Without this stroking, the person will be less trusting and find it difficult to develop confidence in self and others.

Trust, the educators tell us, can be developed later on, but with difficulty. A recent survey, which will be examined in subsequent chapters, reveals that those with trust problems are more likely to get in trouble with substances.

These people are all around us—potentials for addiction. You can see people in your own universe of family and friends who tend to be skeptical, aloof and non-demonstrative about their feelings—they are products of a non-stroking upbringing. As such, they harbor resentments, tend to be loners and suffer along with poor self-image. This is part of what some experts call the "addictive personality." Besides drugs, alcohol, and nicotine, they are likely subjects for obesity, sexual dysfunction, workaholism, disease, and other personal and social maladies.

Another of Erikson's discoveries is that of **industry,** which occurs around four or five years of age and can be seen in how a child goes about finding out how things work. Children who take a watch or clock apart to figure out what makes it tick are examples of industry—they want to know the answers. Why is the moon usually only seen at night? Where does the light go when the switch is flicked? Why, Daddy, why? And other seemingly imponderable questions.

If the child receives responsive answers to endless questions, he or she develops industry, or translated to adult terms, the ability to solve problems. Later on, a girl or boy may apply this skill to bake a cake from scratch. A boy or girl may use it in Little League to hit the cut-off instead of trying to throw directly to the plate to nip a base runner. It's basic training in systems and systems approaches.

Growing up they are unafraid to tackle even the most difficult task because they instinctively know that everything can be figured out. If deprived of this early instinct, the adult can be reticent to get involved in other than minor mysteries. Such a child makes an ideal bureaucrat, doing only what is asked, rather than searching for better ways.

Again, problem solving can be taught but its creative skein is generally very short unless the early development was deep. If disallowed from taking things apart and/or being scolded for doing so, the child learns not to look into matters with any degree of interest or perseverance.

Each of us gains some level of competence on Erikson's continuum of development. The more we absorb as a child, though, the more likely will we use that learning as an adult with growing facility. If we fall into the middle range of development, we'll probably learn some of the skill through experience as an adult, especially if we have a teacher, supervisor, or mentor who figures out what is lacking in the first place. If we are in the lower range of early childhood development, we will certainly have a more difficult time recouping, and in some cases may never achieve other than a modicum of expertise.

Which brings us to how this impacts most on the adolescent. Two of Erickson's stages occur during the teen years; the first is **self identity** and the second is **autonomy.** Combined, they make up the matrix which causes so much turmoil and pain associated with parental and child dysfunction during that period.

Oddly enough, self identity returns to most adults and has come to be called mid-life crisis, which results in career and lifestyle changes, divorce and other chaotic conditions for many Americans.

LIKE THE BEAT, THE SEARCH FOR EXCELLENCE GOES ON

The search for self, who am I, is as common among the rich as the poor, as important to males as females and is the cause for most of the service enterprise in this country. People look to schools, churches, work, clubs, family, friends, the occult, books, seminars, travel, and other means to help discover the "real me." Adolescents, at a time when they are at the greatest risk, also want to know those answers and because of their impatience they want to know right now. **Impatience** is the cultural characteristic given of most young people.

They are involved in that period of growth in which their physical, mental, and emotional as well as spiritual self is at the most steep on the learning curve. They will never experience such growth in their bodies, minds, and feelings as during adolescence. It's fragile period as well—a time when they can upset their own apple carts with a careless experiment here or there. Once they get a whiff of their identity, they want to move on to adulthood even if they are only 12 or 14 years old.

Once they have gained a little knowledge of themselves either by some sense of achievement at school, in sports, or with friends, they feel ready to cut the familial cord. They exhibit this deep-seeded desire for **expression of self** in a variety of ways known intimately by parents from all walks of life.

Simultaneously, they want to be free of restrictions, demanding independence. When they don't get it, they rebel against authority in the most cunning, sometimes overt and sometimes devious ways. Often outrageous, they also can be fiercely protective of their new found identities. They want to be autonomous, but fail to understand that this road is a long one to be traveled many years and features a skill that is honed and chiseled over a lifetime.

Being skilled in **autonomy** is one of the most precarious and vulnerable of Erickson's stages. To be one's own person—the essence of autonomy—is a come-and-go thing in a society where rebels are not easily accepted or adapted into a culture that features more of a "me-too" mentality. The maverick, although idealized in poetry and prose, is seldom welcomed by the majority, which is more in tune with mundane and predictable ways of doing things. The maverick invents, the rest of us utilize it.

Unless, then, the adolescent has been encouraged during these trying times, the instinctive beauty of knowing yourself well enough to know that there's often more to learn, and being able to withstand taunts and pressures from those around you, will go by the boards.

Unfortunately, parents, too, have trouble with these particular stages. They find it worse than the "terrible twos." That's not to blame and isolate the trouble, but to put it into perspective. The elements of the conflict that most mothers and fathers and their offspring go through are centered around **expectations, behaviors,** and **values.** Parents expect the kids, who are not fully grown and certainly not skilled, to behave according to the basic set of values they've been exposed to and are supposedly teaching. Parents can't have it both ways—either the child is an adolescent or not.

Kids, on the other hand, don't know the values as succinctly as do the parents and are operating from their own expectations, and so behave differently—not "good or bad," just differently. They've learned the core values from home, but express them in a different configuration—coded—so the parents can't quite read them readily. Kids are like that.

When these first few conflicts over values go unresolved, the communications deteriorate and the gap of understanding between loved ones gets out of hand. One time the mother may side with the father or child, while in another instance it's vice versa. The resulting confusion from a pattern of "choosing sides" keeps the family from reaching the common goal of having the child grow up in the best fashion possible.

And therein lies the rub because usually in this environment is where drugs, alcohol, and cigarettes become apparent... no pun intended. In some cases, the substance is the target of the conflict and in others it becomes a relief station where the adolescent goes to find solace and comfort. Even in those remote and few cases where relationships within the family are not strained and in chaos, kids in a hurry are likely to experiment with nicotine, booze, and marijuana.

PARADOX OF ADOLESCENCE

Experts tell us that experimentation is the kernel of growth. Without it we don't reach out and stretch to our potential. With it, we fill out and muscle up. Under guidance, and with the exercise of careful thought, kids discover who they are, what they can do, and maybe get an inkling of what they want to be. So with trepidation parents encourage experimentation, hoping that good judgment is used.

But the statistics can be cruel to those parents who want the best for their children. A parent group in Georgia, Parent Resource Institute for Drug Education (PRIDE), surveyed 6,100 seventh graders and found 43% had already tried beer and wine and 23% got intoxicated on hard stuff. The National Council on Alcoholism, Inc. cites 3.3 million drinking teens aged 13 to 17 with difficulties relating to abuse. The trouble ranges from truancy to poor academic performance to the anti-social behaviors of fighting and stealing.

Like the car driver of the opening story, too many teens are mixing booze, drugs, and cigarettes. A couple of tokes on a marijuana joint may not be seen as serious as getting drunk on a six-pack ("...no one's overdosed on marijuana," or so the argument goes), yet the relationship of being stoned, blitzed, blasted, bombed, ripped, etc. is evident. Young people are emulating what they see older people do. While the parents may only drink, or smoke an occasional joint, the foundation is laid for the youngster to try it. And in many cases want to do them one better. The American way is to want to outperform one's parents.

Even if the household is not where they see adults behave familiarly with substance, the temptation to try one, the other, or all three is huge. It's on television, in the movies, in cartoons, and in every possible known media. They hear about it from their best, or worst, friends. The allure is as persistent as any advertising campaign designed by a competent behavioral scientist—try this and you'll get as high as you've ever been, and quicker, too.

You get high, that's for sure, but the low is a bummer. What goes up, must come down, according to the lyrics of the old nursery rhyme. With drugs, the bottom is a sewer of trouble.

AND YET ANOTHER COUNTY HEARD FROM

Acquired Immune Defiency Syndrome (AIDS) is one of the troubles. AIDS is frequently transmitted through dirty needles of drug users, according to medical authorities. AIDS a fatal disease for which no cure is available, was once thought to be solely prevalent amongst homosexuals. Not so. It's also transmitted in blood transfusions. You get AIDS and you're in a life-threatened situation.

The deaths in 1986 of professional athletes Len Bias, former Maryland basketball player who had just signed a multi-million dollar deal with the world champion Boston Celtics, and Don Rogers, defensive halfback of the Cleveland Browns from Sacramento, highlighted another **"you do drugs and you die"** scenario. These deaths touched off a national awareness and education flurry that raised a national consciousness. What remained to be done was how do we get our kids to stop, or better yet, not get started.

Bias and Rogers allegedly snorted cocaine and suffered the consequences. Cocaine is serious business and deaths directly attributed to its use rose 325% in 1986 according to the Drug Enforcement Administration (DEA), a federal agency within the Justice Department. A 37% rise in Emergency Room admissions and deaths were cocaine-related. Repeated cocaine use causes nasal and other respiratory damage akin to pouring hydrochloric acid in your face. "Coke" is a high risk drug.

The coke derivative, crack, is now an additional threat to young people because it's relatively cheap and easy to obtain. Besides more addictive than coke, crack is also more erractic in chemical content and far more dangerous to the health of the user. Because it has similar potency of freebasing without the inconvenience, it's the current lure. In other words, you don't even have to be addicted to get hurt from this stuff.

In addition some half million heroin addicts are in this country, a portion of whom are in treatment on either methadone or naxlythone. Because both treatments are addictive, the patient gets off one drug onto to another, a cycle that keeps the addict in chains.

Designer drugs, which are produced by altering the molecular structure of a wide variety of compounds, can increase potency by 150 to 1,000 times. These synthetics can virtually leave the person paralyzed in his or her own body. A little knowledge of chemistry can go a long way to chop your head off. It's the modern version of "Dr. Jekyl and Mr. Hyde."

And now to marijuana. Like drinkers and smokers, it has its share of user proponents. They put out the claim that moderation prevents the person from being addicted and this is usually supported with scientific evidence. Nonetheless, it is a significant contributor to large pockets of poor health in America.

SOME MEDICAL EVIDENCE

In a pamphlet published by the National Organization for the Reform of Marijuana Laws (NORML), it says one of the chemicals in marijuana, Delta 9 THC, produces a psychoactive effect. Smoke from a reefer irritates the lungs and heavy exposure increases the likelihood of lung cancer and other lung problems. Likewise, marijuana speeds the heartbeat and is unhealthy for people with high blood pressure or other cardiovascular diseases.

Marijuana reduces the sperm count and obstructs sperm mobility in males. Because it crosses the placenta, like other drugs, NORML advises pregnant women to avoid using it.

Others, however, make hard medical claims against the reefer. Most of the 30 million regular users of marijuana smoke it. Some make Alice B Toklas brownies or muffins, but in the main it is ingested as a cigarette. Smoking cigarettes of normal tobacco is hazardous enough to one's health—it's more so with marijuana with its 421 chemicals.

Medical experts say it causes brain damage, reduces motivation, is a driving safety hazard, and does other psychological and biological damage, especially to adolescents who are much more susceptible to such imbalances than adults. While much of the definitive data is scientifically inconclusive about marijuana, enough is out to arouse parents of elementary and junior high school pupils.

Those against marijuana use/abuse link it to higher order drugs as the next step in the addiction process. A user of marijuana for ten years recently told his counselor, *"I'm not an addict. But I would find it very hard to give up smoking dope. I just enjoy it too much."*

While the prohibitionists use some exaggeration in their claims against the ill effects of grass, their collective voice has kept marijuana high on the list of crimes in this nation, mainly because of the purported medical problems associated with it.

THE ECONOMICS OF IT

In a previously mentioned Baltimore study of drugs and crime, what is apparent is that users and abusers need a lot of money to support their habits. Drugs in this country are beyond

Big Business—it's Mega Business. Depending on the source, it's between $80 billion and $150 billion a year enterprise. In California, it's the largest cash crop. Nationally, it's in second place by only a whisker of corn.

The nation spends a lot of money on the supply side of the drug problem. Marijuana prohibition, for example, amounts to $5 billion at the federal, state, and local level, with dubious results. Of that the federal outlay in 1986 was $2 billion, most of which was for new border agents and a few international agents. The result of that in "busts" amounted to about $2 billion, including cocaine and other imported illicit drugs.

For the feds it was a push. But that's not even a draw between all the good guys and bad guys. Besides you can't be sure of the accuracy of the economics of the busts because of multiple claims—federal, state, and local law enforcement agencies don't do well on working together and often vie for media attention. So a certain amount of claim jumping occurs.

These busts cost a lot. The cost of arresting people is high. Since 1970, more than five million Americans have been busted on marijuana charges, mainly for possession. Of the 410,000 arrested annually on marijuana charges, 85% are for possession, not dealing. In contrast, only about half that number, 200,000 Americans, were arrested for rape, robbery, and murder combined.

The marijuana laws do little for rehabilitation. Not much is built into the education and reorientation aspect of the "crime." One study revealed the 94% of dope users continued to do so after being arrested and many continue to smoke even while in prison. It's either a sin or it isn't. We've got to make up our societal mind and do more than a collective tsk-tsk.

These sins of commission against society, and perhaps against even higher authority, continue despite growing alarm and money being thrown at the epidemic. Personal debilitation wreaks havoc at home, work, and school. Dr. Mark Gold, who instituted the 800-Cocaine Hotline four years ago, found that a huge sample of users agree that they function at 67% of peak efficiency after drug use. They accelerate temporarily while stoned, but fall off dramatically, often needing another hit to feel "together."

Dr. Gold also reports drug users suffer a 350% higher chance of an accident than non-users. Workers' compensation claims are five times higher for drug users than non, and they tend to use employee benefits three times more than other employees. Straight corporate employees are subsidizing their doper co-workers.

When Dr. Gold set up his service to help those who sought it, he expected to hear from about 10,000 people a year. Imagine his surprise to receive 1,200 calls each and every day—then and since.

His callers have the opportunity to receive answers to perplexing facets of the trouble—how do I detect if someone is using, what are the symptoms, how harmful is it, what can I do about it for myself, my kids, or my spouse? They also are asked to answer questions for Dr. Gold's data base on use, abuse, costs, performance, productivity, availability, safety, and related aspects. These answers are not heartening.

Of the 1,200 who call every day, 75% are users—900 a day. Of them, 92% use on the job or, if students, at school. Some 64% admit to poor performance as a result and nearly two in five said they would use more if they had the money. One fourth of the callers use daily and nearly half are weekend "recreational" users—a term that has meaning only in the media...medical sources insist use is use and no glamourizing modifier will soften the impact of cocaine addiction.

Three of every four users is habitually late to work, meetings, and other appointments and one-half of the callers have dealt to others to keep their own supply intact. Nearly one-third have lost their jobs or have come close to it because of their addiction to cocaine. A surprising number, 64%, said they would use more often if it were available.

Cocaine is the Yuppie drug of choice. One DEA sample indicated the cocaine addict is male (82%), age 31, earning

$83,000 a year and snorting $1,500 a week. But look at the pipeline—the feeder system for future Yuppies. Adolescents from the same survey are spending $440 a week on their habit; 43% are in debt; 42% have dealt the drug to keep their supply alive; 38% steal to pay for it; 33% suffered poor performance and related problems in school; 18% have been suspended once, and 20% have been arrested.

Of those surveyed, only 65% felt addicted, yet 85% were unable to turn it down when it was available or offered to them for sale. In terms of choice, 60% preferred it to food, 50% to friends, 68% to family, and 35% took coke over sex.

Those in the know about cocaine believe this is only the tip of the iceberg. A high tech connection exists—people who work with their heads believe drugs help their non-linear thinking capabilities. The rationalization is that the risk of addiction is worth the few moments of altered mind state.

Even in absence of pre-existing family problems, the drug does its best to turn father against child, child against sibling, and ruin what God intended to be a home of comfort, caring, and growth.

William F. Alden, chief of the DEA, pointed out that drugs, whether legal or not, comprise most of the Emergency Room (ER) admissions in American hospitals today. One-half of the ER admissions are related to legally prescribed drugs, such as tranquilizers, barbiturates, amphetamines, and others. You know them as valium, sleeping pills, speed, uppers, and so on.

Alden cited statistics that show 20 million Americans use legally prescribed drugs for non-medical reasons—a white collar criminal scenario of mammoth proportions. And you don't read much about that in today's news spotlight on drugs.

Illegally manufactured drugs such as PCP, LSD, and others crop into the news and become attractive for prostitutes, burglars, and other street criminals. These criminals, Alden reminded us, once were just kids who started to have trouble in adolescence.

He told of some gains—heroin use has been stabilized in the past five years—but a new version, "black tar" from Mexico, is responsible for a 100% increase in ER admissions. Heroin becomes the base for the so-called designer drugs. As noted earlier, it's relatively easy to set up a laboratory and get into business making synthetics.

TOO MANY COOKS IN THE KITCHEN?

So what's being done about the addiction problem in this country?

Well, for one thing the Reagan Administration started a War on Drugs, which began in 1984 with the Comprehensive Crime Bill, giving focus to federal, state, and local enforcement officials. This was strengthened by the Anti-Drug Abuse Act signed into existence in 1986 by President Reagan.

Interdiction has been stepped up with the addition of several hundred agents bringing the total up to 2,700 in 1986. The Coast Guard uses its planes and ships in efforts to thwart smugglers on land, air, and sea, coming from Columbia, Mexico, the Mediteranean countries, and elsewhere. Narcotics specialists are trained to infiltrate organized crime groups in efforts to locate the "connections" through which the drug traffic flows.

You can't turn on the television without a special program on ABC, NBC, CBS, and the cable networks discussing the sordid and costly aspects of drug abuse. Books, movies, video cassettes, seminars, workshops, and lectures focus on the dilemma. They pile on the statistics and you can hear the collective "tsk, tsk" resound from school group to church group to juvenile halls throughout the country.

Police officers take to the school room to talk "straight" with kids and some even get their parents to sit in on some sessions. In Los Angeles, Project DARE funds five officers to conduct 17-week programs covering self esteem, self worth, and problem solving—all with a core theme of drugs and the harm it does.

Treatment programs abound, too. Tough Love, founded in Texas by a church group, offers a family-oriented approach to support kids wanting to kick the habit. States like California, Massachusetts, Illinois, Georgia, New York, and others have pilot programs for young criminal offenders with an alcohol and drug problem. Some cities like Houston, Texas and Concord, California have police involved with private consultants to work with first-time offending adolescents and their families. (One of these will be examined in greater detail later.)

And it's somewhat frightening to hear that 60 airline pilots are under treatment, 10% of all the big city bus drivers, and who knows how many truck drivers who regularly pound their five-ton and more rigs down heavily trafficked highways across this land of ours. Treatment takes care of some who have, in essence, been caught or turned themselves in. At least it gets some off the travel byways and highways.

Yet, when you examine the statistical trends, nothing seems to be getting better. In some categories, like heroin abuse, the numbers are somewhat stabilized, although you can talk to those in the treatment arena and they don't find any let up. In other categories, such as qualudes, a reduction in supply appears to be occurring. In all other areas, the demand side of the equation seems unaffected. With all the attention, tv commercials, booklets by the thousands, and talk, the problem remains.

Some say a national strategy is needed to combine the turf competition amongst federal, state, and local agencies so that all can focus on the various aspects—a czar of drugs to set the agenda and allocate resources.

But will that get to the 25% of Rockwell International employees who tested positive for drugs? (Rockwell is one of the country's largest space and defense contractors.) That's not to pick on Rockwell—many companies who could qualify too for such a listing. The computer-related industries and departments within medium and low tech industries seem to be most suspect for drug abuse. Alcoholism makes little or no distinction when it comes to work sites.

The question is can you imagine another government agency trying to coordinate with the 37 others at the federal level alone and then getting the 50 states and 1,500 municipalities to go along? What ever happened to president Reagan's well-intentioned and ambitious program to cut down the size of federal bureacracy? It's too bad we just can't start over with a new deck and play the game.

ANY PROGRESS IN SIGHT?

The recovery rate of addicts is low, while the recitivism rate is high. Once the pattern is established, it's very difficult to alter. Not impossible, just very difficult. Once a young man or woman goes to prison for drug-related crimes, nine out of ten will return to the criminal activity. Most will be caught again and returned. Some gains new skills while incarcerated, making it more difficult for apprehension when they get out.

Alcoholics Anonymous tells its multi-million members that they will always be alcoholics, albeit recovering ones. But the lure to return to the bottle is great. If the cause is not dealt with, the pain may well return. The drink eases the hurt and as one way says, "You don't drown your troubles, you merely teach them to swim." Similarly, once a dopester has been sent sky high by a snort of this or an injection of that, he or she experiences an ecstasy seldom enjoyed through natural means. At least not as quickly.

So they fall off the wagon when the pressure of the job or the strain of school gets to them. They seek out old places and haunts where drugs are commonplace and the rituals of camaraderie can be practiced with jovial, though costly routines. They aren't "addicts" but they can't seem to kick the habit. A commonly heard phrase in those distant, lonely corners is *"God help me."*

Maybe that is the only answer. Maybe it's beyond human skills to get at the bottom of this. Maybe it's the curse of the evil empire. Or, maybe the solution has been covered up with all the media emphasis on how severe the supply side condition is...maybe the answer is just beneath the surface of all the hype.

FOCUS ON PREVENTION

A new survey of more than 200 families, counselors, addicts, law officials, teachers, and others involved in thinking about prevention puts the focus on lifestyle education. Not traditional education of a teacher or irate parent poking a finger at a kid and repeating some myth or partial truth. The education that will work this time involves:

- accurate research,
- a forum for sensible talk amongst the concerned parties,
- a measurement of progress, and
- enough time for the process to take root.

It will need nurturing and caring for. It will be family-based. That's what the survey respondents said.

In interviews with parents, for example, they often were unaware of how far along their adolescent child was in the drug scene. *"Oh, I knew Jill had taken a few drinks. Hell, we have it here at the house all the time. But LSD? That blew our minds. I just don't know how one kid could turn out that way when the others are so straight."*

Others said, *"Drugs can sure cause a lot of physical damage to the body that I didn't know about. Had I known I'm sure I'd have taken better precautionary means to watch for signs. I just didn't know how dangerous these damn things can be."*

Or, *"Why didn't the school do more to get us involved? I'm busy, sure, but I'd have taken the time to learn about the seriousness of this drug business. I think that I'd even do a little about cutting down on my bad habits of drinking and smoking. I'm sure I would if the schools had forced me to attend some sessions."*

One of the surprises of the survey was that many parents felt ill-equipped to teach the good, old time, basic values and were not reluctant to turn the responsibility over to the beleagured schools. The schools, unfortunately, consider their job more in terms of texts and content than character building.

"There's not enough time nor money to get heavily into drug prevention or intervention," said a vice principal at a

Northern California school noted for its quality scholastic and athletic record. Jack Keegan wryly added, *"We don't teach family . . . and I wish we could. We have a Students Against Drunk Driving (SADD) chapter and they do a variety of activities to involve the community, parents, kids, church groups, law enforcement and others in a year-long program of education."* It helps.

Keegan's implication was that parents seemed most reticent of all the people to want to face up to the reality of the drinking and drug epidemic facing their progeny. Maybe it's because they don't believe it could happen to their family. That's a major part of their reluctance, according to the survey. Another drawback is the down-the-road possibility that they'd have to change a little, and that's uncomfortable when you've worked so hard to gain some stability and comfort in your life. Nonetheless, it keeps many parents from greater involvement.

Then, too, they are busy with their own professional and social lives. Work comes first with most. Business pays the bills and provides the amenities and luxuries all the family enjoys. Why else would Dad (or Mom, in more and more cases as dual career couples and single parent families grow in number) work hard and long hours? This is more than a rhetorical query, which will be answered in part in Chapter 5. And, after family comes friends.

A FRIEND IN NEED

My grandfather used to say, *"You can always tell the character of someone by the friends he or she keeps."* Gramps wasn't any intellectual genius but contemporary authority and conventional wisdom seem to agree. The term they use is "peer pressure" to describe why kids do anything wrong. The research bears out some of this "truth" as many adolescents admit that a friend talked, cajoled, or bribed them into their first drink, cigarette, joint, or pill.

No one held a gun to their head, forcing them into action yet most of these dubious invitations are accepted if it comes from a friend. What are friends for, anyway?

Friendship always comes in second, on average, to family as the most powerful guider of values in our society. A fair percentage of young people score friends ahead of mom, pop, and siblings when it comes to providing a soft shoulder and open ear. So goes it in the perplexing times of growing up.

So even in those times when it would be best to sound out family members for a problem, often they happen to be unsympathetic, too busy, or just not available, which is frequently the case. If not family members, then a friend in need, is a friend indeed.

Friendships made in teen years often are the most durable, lasting a lifetime. A recent AT&T television commercial theme pointed this out as the oldtimer recalls childhood incidents and calls the friend to reminisce. A beer commercial picks up on the same theme as a group of Yuppie males discuss their fun days of yesterday over a round of suds. Friends make and often break you, if you let them.

A new television theme, fortunately, picked on the positive aspects of friendship and showed one drinking friend giving up the car keys to another, for friendship's sake. Other friendship themes are portrayed in drug and cigarette prohibition scenes as well. The power of friendship can't be overlooked when prevention comes to mind.

UNITED WE STAND

Nor can the power of the corporation, association, agency, or well-intentioned group when you study the intricacies of keeping loved ones healthy. Many corporations in America—35% of FORTUNE'S 500—have instigated drug testing procedures for hiring and firing employees at all levels. Personnel officials in the private and public sectors claim such efforts have clamped down on drug use by 30% to 50%. These urine tests, however, have created a storm of controversy which will be examined more fully in Chapter 9. Testing looms large as one facet of a total prevention package, especially in the corporate world. It's going to scare some people off drugs.

Schools, where the administration, board, and teachers' union work together, have also acquitted themselves well on the prevention issue despite limited time and funds. Their focus, however, has created opposition because of the legal ramifications and the imperfect measurement system. Many teachers, though, find the hassle of confronting a child on what looks to be a drug problem, too much to handle.

Irate parents, non-supportive administrators, arrogant lawyers and tearful youngsters pose a condition unconducive for many. Only in schools where a coordinated and integrative approach is taken to involve the school board, the union, the administration, parent groups, and a trained teacher cadre is success guaranteed to cut and curb the use by pupils. Even in these ideal situations, the cure is often more painful than continuation. Some advocates of a drug-free society are uncomfortable with the fear tactics used to curb individual freedom. And then the inevitable occurs. Kids continue to do drugs and risk suspension, arrest, and isolation from friends and peers.

While testing can impact on some people using marijuana, it misses other drugs which cause more impairment. It also is not flawless in picking out weed smokers. People wrongly judged as drug users can and have sued for millions. Opponents of urine testing point to an emergence of a new drug-testing industry replete with drug counselors, unprecedented growth in the drug treatment business, and, they claim, the risk of a cheating industry which will evolve to get faked reports for the tested individual. None of which really does much to get at the heart of the matter—why do drugs in the first place?

TO THINE OWN SELF BE TRUE

Experts in the people business—sociologists, psychiatrists, ministers, counselors, educators, and others—have come to a consensus on the conceptual solution, which is for increased self-awareness by those who haven't used, and lifestyle change for those who have.

Jon B. Gettman, national director of NORML, says educational programs have successfully reduced the number of nicotine addicts in America and increased the number of seat belt wearers. He and his organization advocate similar efforts ".. . to educate the public about marijuana, the marijuana laws, and their effect on society. It's our contention that the project of discouraging marijuana use is better handled by education than law enforcement."

Self-awareness through education is the first step to eradication of any societal problem. The trouble is that misinformation and disinformation is harder to separate from factual data than taking fly droppings from the pepper. One school of thought is invariably contested by another equally funded, researched and vigorous. The stalemate seems interminable. Each axe to be ground takes the wheel from another grinder. The ox that is gored is at the expense of another farmer. What generally happens in our litigious country is that the argument goes to court with only a temporary judgement, and in many cases, it's the lawyers who win the most.

If health is a central issue to the argument, how healthy can we get. Diet books are among the highest selling in the book stores and book clubs. Either people soon forget what they read or fail to maintain their initial interest and motivation. The ray of hope is that after ten years of media hype on personal health, nearly 70 million Americans have taken it upon themselves to take better care of their health through exercise, nutrition, and relaxation. This way of coping with a world filled with anxiety and stress has its benefits seen in trimmer bodies, altered lifestyles, and longevity.

Dr. Meyer Friedman, co-author of the book on Type A behavior, recently released new information on how counseling, diet, exercise, and relaxation reduced by one-half the cardiovascular difficulties of heart attack victims. The premise is that given a system to follow, people will adapt their behavior. While Mike Friedman doesn't advertise it, his program also includes a hefty dose of spirituality.

While the video version of Jane Fonda helps millions "go for the burn" to get in physical shape, hundreds of writers and essayists from Norman Vincent Peale to Edgar Cayce to Marilyn Ferguson bring attention to the need for emotional, mental, and spiritual discipline in daily life. This is the Age of Aquarius!

Each guru has a different and unique twist and turn and offers food for thought. Those dealing specifically with addiction talk and write about an integrative approach, yet their systems haven't yet made much progress on this multi billion-dollar destruction. Somebody's listening, though.

Where is the leakage occurring? What part of the pie slips out of the neatly constructed theory and allows the adolescent to experiment beyond his or her means to handle it? The format for good behavior is the same as for bad habits. You become aware of the experience, check your attitude about it, and then bounce it off your value system to make a judgment about keeping at it. If your tracking system is not flawed, you keep going.

Having a clear perspective of one's tracking system seems to be the problem with adolescents. They may know at one level—physical, emotional, intellectual, or spiritual—that doing drugs, drinks, and cigarettes is wrong for them, but they rarely realize it simultaneously at all four. Well, neither do many adults.

ONE FOR ALL, ALL FOR ONE

The multi-disciplinary, systems approach to life is only now beginning to catch on in America. We're slowly shedding the specialization era that was fostered by Henry Ford in industrial America and by John Dewey in education. We're on the brink of valuing the integrative quality of life. The Japanese and even the reluctant Europeans have learned that collaboration works better than internal competitiveness. Competition, they say, is for goal-setting and the external groups.

Although it's often argued by scholars that the founding fathers, who gave equal opportunity to all its citizens, intended an integrated society, the separationists of church and state muddied up the intention. Life on earth was ordained to be integrated, not segmented as some would have you believe. The idea of harmony, justice, truth, beauty, and love cannot be considered without integration. The product of segmentation, separation, and isolation is seen in addiction.

American coins all have three similarities. Each has the words Liberty, In God We Trust, and E Pluribus Unum stamped on them. Our paper money is less similar (and often as volatile in world economic markets) as only In God We Trust is consistently imprinted—Liberty and E Pluribus Unum have vanished. One can make the conjecture that, while God maintains a general economic appeal, the citizenry is less concerned with unity and freedom. Of course, that's not the intention, but one could argue the point.

Recent court decisions in Tennessee and Texas, for example, have allowed that God, in form of a Supreme Being, Universal Energy, or other designation, can be part of some texts, providing equal opportunity is given to other possibilities for creation and a natural order of things. Does this gnaw at the fabric of our Constitution? Few doubt it, although, as previously mentioned, some opposition will likely evolve to take the other side. Ours is an adversarial culture.

A CRUSADE LOOKING FOR CRUSADERS

The War on Drugs is a serious one. It's big money, meaning serious. But money won't win it. Look at Viet Nam. We spent more than we did during World Wars I and II combined and had to leave without a victory. Despite the fact that 58,000 American youths died there, the will of the people fighting for their own country overcame our vast military might and money. Critics argued that it would have been cheaper to buy the land than to wage war against people fighting for their right to live where they've always lived. It would have surely raised their standard of living.

To win the war against addiction it will take a fervor akin to a religious war. It will take more than a nodding intellectualization that "sure, it's serious and I'll pay my taxes to see it won." It requires more than the emotional agony of parents and families whose youngsters have fallen to addiction. If the physical pain of the addicted could be channeled to the battle, it would not be enough. And, sadly stated, praying to God will not end the devastation.

Each element of society already involved should be enough to put the problem to rest, but it hasn't and won't. It will take a crusade with all facets working in harmony with the others to end the pain, corruption, and suffering. And it won't require a czar.

Nowadays people are pretty sophisticated and are not likely to embrace that concept easily. You can hear the kibitzers. *"Me dress up in a uniform and march somewhere? Not likely. I don't look good in armored mail."*

"I'm really not that religious and even if I was, I doubt my church/synagogue/sect would go along with such an idea."

The jesters and skeptics would rally around for a field day that would put Babylon to the third class seats by comparison. Is our society so steeped in materialism and hedonism? The evidence points otherwise. A growing group of health-seekers and change-makers is emerging in companies, churches, schools, government, and other institutions. More importantly, the advocates for better-living-through-less-chemistry are looking inward first, and to their own new and growing families second—a rapid one-two punch.

They find precedence in a variety of places. They read about systems and their effectiveness in their work. They see it at work in government coalitions. They see old barriers being broken down between long-standing foes like the U.S. and China, Egypt and Israel, and such on the global scene. The mergers of former competitors in the computer, transportation, and other industrial situations are a strong indication that previously held animosities can be withdrawn and the energies can be redirected toward more suitable goals. They can read it, too, in the Bible—old and new testament versions. **A synergy of forces can yield outcomes necessary for short- and long-term gains.**

THE CRUSADER SYSTEM—21st CENTURY STYLE

Crusaders of olden days began their struggle with an idea that the Holy Grail could be found, they would gain salvation in the process and that the world would be a better place than when they started. These ideals are not a bad place to start this new crusade.

In this instance, the Holy Grail is a country free of dependency on drugs, alcohol, and cigarettes. The infusion of a new spirit will be a salvation of a different kind to those who get involved—a security in knowing their children will be free to grow to their fullest without internal restrictions. With that in mind, the world can only be a better place than the drugged culture in which we now live.

The system, while simple, will take time to be learned and then more time will be necessary for full-term growth. How long is difficult to say. Maybe a year, maybe two, but probably three to five years for the learning. Maybe a generation for full-term growth.

It's three parts are simple enough: Alpha, Beckoning, and Crusade.

Alpha is the start, the beginning. It's also the brightest star in the galaxy and the first word in the Greek alphabet. It is here that you start. With a bright light, you begin your assessment of the current reality. An assessment can be made of the personal human condition in terms of basic values—the forces that drive and energize people. Then look at what tools or skills the individual has, what shape they are in, and what needs to be done to get them in better working order. The last part of Alpha or assessment is a close look at the opportunities for success whether for yourself, your friends, and/or family members.

Alpha is the starting place. To begin a journey, you must first know where you are. While this sounds obvious, many people merely guess at or assume they know their location, the condition of the vehicle, the shape of the roads, and the weather forecast. Assessment is not to be confused with procrastination. It is another word for stage one in planning.

Once you've looked inside and found some fundamental information, you engage the second gear, which is Beckoning. **Beckoning** is the allure of the quest—the promise of the effort, the joy and glory of achievement. If you turn the engine on and it roars to life, you engage the gears and feel a natural energy release and aim it for the distant star. Beckoning is energy, power, and adventure in the highest sense. It combines your will with a new direction for your thoughts, feelings, and being.

This uplifting experience takes place which begin to sharpen the tools you have and put them to work on cutting away dead wood and clear the ground for planting new seeds. You enlist others in the preparation and they catch your contagious energy. Passions become reality with a fixed and soft focus on wonderful new and in-reach horizons.

Learning replaces out-dated tapes and a spring comes to your step and the environment. Conflict is replaced with clarity, confusion becomes opportunity, doubt turns into easy rhythm and harmony. Science merges with art, the teacher becomes student and hate turns to love. This comes to be through action. Insight from Alpha lends itself to vigorous ventures into new lands. Risk taking is broadened and growth builds confidence and strength, enabling a young person to stand TALL—the posture of a crusader.

This brings the **crusader** to the heart of the matter. A commitment to this new way of living. The trust in God on the coin becomes a personal trust, a path to follow. The Crusade is the third and ongoing stage—the process of nature. Being more a part of what God intended is what the Crusade is all about. Nothing can top this way of putting forth yourself. It's a connection of Alpha and Beckoning to change yourself first and then joining others who have chosen similarly.

The system is quite easy and productive. It's not always simple and at times you may experience great turmoil. It may scare you and you may think you've failed. But that's only part of the process. it's normal to be apprehensive and impatient. As you learn your way, you'll feel newfound joy and energy. As you track your progress, you'll wonder why you didn't do this sooner.

SUMMARY

Addiction is a national tragedy, which continues despite tons of money being poured at the problem. The costs are not economic alone—people who are addicted are in pain, their friends and family suffer, and they are a societal loss.

Adolescence is the time to enhance life, not stunt it. More can be done to help young, impatient people grow up.

The emphasis on curtailing supply is necessary but not at the cost of educating and arming young people, their parents, and teachers. A business as large as drug trafficking is not going to die slowly. Like buggy whips, though, it can shrivel up because the horse of a different color shows up.

Prevention is the best cure. Prevention is a system that is comprised of assessment, action and commitment in a physical, emotional, intellectual, and spiritual way—a synergistic solution to the addiction and health dilemma in America, a way to stand TALL as a crusader.

Chapter **2**

NO IS NOT ENOUGH

As he dressed for the sail club meeting, Tommy Ward overheard his mother talking with her sister, Aunt Helen. He shook his head and wondered why she always did that; why did Mom always say one thing and do another.

"You wouldn't believe it, Hel," she was saying. "I don't know why I went to that outrageously expensive store in the first place. The sale, I suppose. I browsed and browsed. You know what a good browser I am. I bought a scarf for Bette's birthday, a couple of do dads for the house, and then I saw this elegant pants suit. Linen. Carmel with gold and silver piping. Beautiful cut. Those fashionable oversized shoulders. Of course, it wasn't on sale. Cost a fortune. Honest, Hel, I don't know why I bought it but I wanted it and . . ."

Tommy walked through, waving goodbye to Aunt Helen and his mother. He carried the sailing charts under his arm as he half-walked, half-ran toward the meeting; he wondered why his mother did that. It didn't seem right. And what was wrong with Dad? Lately, he'd come home for supper, hit the bottle for a couple of drinks or more, and falls asleep on the couch, sometimes before eating or right after. Boy, what was happening with my folks.

What influence does the indulgent mother and overindulgent father have on a 16-year-old, nearing the finish of his own special period of growth and choice? He's changing rapidly. Going from Cub Scout blue to Sea Scout blue is only one alteration in reality. He'll be seeking the new highs associated with adolescence...the thrills of youth...the freedom for action.

This scene and many like it in America pose a societal dysfunction that plays a part in the substance abuse problem. The Ward family has two healthy parents, a healthy son and, on the surface, a healthy home life. Just beneath the calm, though, they face a treacherous undercurrent—a disease is festering.

Each of the members seems vaguely aware of his or her status. No deep questioning exists of the malaise; only ritual behavior that drugs the conscious mind. No one senses that a valued potential is being wasted. They are living out banal scripts, not the ones given to them as a birthright in this country.

For Walt and Ellen, it's an arguable point of contention. We don't really have enough data about them. Almost in passing they seem like a backdrop against which Tommy Ward grows up. But what about Tommy? He's 16—not a boy, not a man—with a whole life ahead of him.

MORE THAN BLOOD OUT OF A TURNIP

Potential is an elusive concept and equally elusive as a practice. People the world over search for truth, beauty, and goodness at work, at home, in churches, in social settings, and in relationships. Some get close, a few reach it, but most of us fall short. In many cases, those that get close see the opportunity once or twice but for some crazy reason, back away at the last moment. It may seem too real, too frightening, or too mystical for our temporal minds.

Tapping into one's potential can be a frightening thing. It's a twilight zone, foreboding and unknown. The first time we notice our potential generally occurs in adolescence.

A CASE HISTORY

Jenni Jardine quickly crossed the street and took two steps at a time to the front door, pulled it open, avoided looking at the receptionist and headed straight for the women's restroom. *"What is happening?"* she asked herself in quiet horror as she sat on the restroom toilet, examining herself.

She was described by people the last few years as "the girl next door." Perky, studious and dependable were adjectives that fit. Just the kind of daughter anyone would love to have. Jenni had a nice word for everyone and only once in a while did this junior high schooler fly off the handle, losing control of her emotional balance. Today was one of those days. She was bleeding and didn't know what to make of it.

Her mind raced. What did she do recently that could have caused this devastation? Nothing strenuous. She had been feeling, well, grumpy the past few days but she had a lot on her mind—school, the club activities, the tension at home with mom and dad arguing so much, and Tommy Ward's sudden interest in her. Through her tears, she tried to figure out what to do and nothing seemed to make sense.

Later, talking with her friend Tina, they both doubled with laughter as Jenni described how she folded nearly one-half of a roll of toilet paper and stuffed it into her panties as a first aid treatment for her trouble. *"I can't believe you didn't know about your cycle,"* Tina shouted through her laughing. *"I just can't believe it!"*

Embarrassed as she was earlier, Jenni felt relieved but gradually a sense of resentment overcome her. *"Why didn't Mom warn me about this ... it's so ... terrible!"* she thought as she went over the situation in her mind. *"What was it Tina called it—my monthly cycle. Oh, how horrible!"*

Unpleasant though it was, Jenni later shared her anger with her mother and together they had one of the best mother/daughter talks in their lives. Mother assumed that the school's hygiene class had covered the female menstrual condition. She meant to talk with Jenni about it on several occasions, but somehow never did. She apologized, hugged her daughter and both cried happy tears.

It could have been worse. Jenni could have harbored the resentment into adulthood and the conflict between mother and daughter would have widened, probably never to be resolved and never to be understood. Such is the way of relationships.

What Jenni's mother did do, though, was to seize the opportunity to get further into her daughter's development. Mrs. Jardine had been under severe pressure the last two years with her marriage and was not paying the kind of attention to Jenni that she needed and wanted. But now she used the "monthly cycle" as the way to hold ongoing friendly but informative talks about other natural cycles that occur in life.

GETTING ON WITH BALANCING

Nearly all professionals understand that balance, harmony, and rhythm are fundamental to success, yet few professionals in the business, academic and government communities do much about it except, maybe, on a personal level.

Some people are born with good balance, others have to work continuously at developing it. In either case, attention is required to keep it once you've got it. Because no one gets out of this life alive, it becomes a matter of life and death. The person who learns the secret of harmony will be more successful, enjoy life and its rhythm, and be more attuned to others. Such a person has the earmarks of a warrior, a crusader, one standing TALL.

Conversely, the out-of-balance individual generally is victimized, or victimizes, causing more pain and grief than the balanced person. And, by virtue of that description, is likely to die sooner.

Dr. William Westerlin Anderson, a native of Rockford, Illinois, grew up in the Midwest, went to school there and began his practice as a neurologist. He didn't quit learning once out of school. He continued studying nerves and then added bone and muscle to his practice of getting patients back in balance. A part of his education was a trip to Japan to watch doctors there manipulate bodies using the triumvirate, and synergistic, theory of nerve, bone, and muscle.

"This is my third innominate rotation of the morning," he explained in his folksy way as he worked to loosen a patient's hamstring muscle so the large pelvic bone and associated tissue

would rotate back into place where it belonged. The patient had "thrown out his back" after an especially stressful couple of weeks. What actually happened was that the stress accumulated and tightened the hamstrings, which pushed the innominate bone out of place.

"*In some cases, the combination of bone, muscle, and tissue can be literally connected to tight hamstrings, setting up a painful back dislocation,*" Dr. Anderson explained. The good doctor knew how to manipulate the thigh muscle to work the bone back in place. He also knows what every school child does— the foot bone's connected to the leg bone, the leg bone's connected to the knee bone, et cetera.

People tend to get out of whack and do themselves all sorts of trouble by allowing stress to remain on their bodies. Dr. Anderson, who now has a private practice in San Mateo and Redwood City, knows the concept of balance and has the medical experience and manipulative tricks to help his patients regain that body harmony. He feels that the Orientals are much further along, as a society, in taking care of themselves as far as balance and harmony go—they come from a synergistic culture.

WHAT IS A CRUSADER?

Men and women of all descriptions can become crusaders. Most Americans have the potential because we evolved from hardy stock, the kind of pioneering person who withstood the adversities of nature. One myth, though, about our ancestors is that they actually conquered nature. This is an illusion . . . because crusaders don't conquer nature, they abide by it.

People who go around trying to conquer nature generally wind up on Dr. Anderson's treatment table, in hospitals, mental wards, or simply beside themselves. Crusaders live within the environment of nature and assist in cleaning up the messes that some human animals make of it. They, too, understand the concept of balance.

A definition of a crusader: **A crusader is one who believes in the natural order of things, develops a dedication to its** *purpose without being single-minded and is respectful of those who also work for harmony.*

That sounds simple enough but it seems to toss many aspirants for the proverbial loop when they try to carry it out in today's pressure-cooker society. Concepts are not easy to put in practice especially with a lot of distractions around. One of the keys to harmony is understanding the historical perspective of the crusader and your relation to it.

A mini-history of America tells the story of hardy pioneers who took on the unknown and settled this country from coast to coast, Mexico to Canada. They didn't settle nature, per se, but they did become settled on one physical part of it. This took a variety of life skills and motivational values—similar to those to be described later in greater detail. These core values and synergy skills are not strangers to America. These crusaders have a historical perspective dating back to the successful pioneer—a connection of history to the present. Sometimes the heritage doesn't surface until we've lived a little and have had some experience under our belts.

SOMETIMES, MOTHER KNOWS BEST

Shirley Jardine was a late bloomer. She had a few friends in high school, tried out for cheerleaders but was not selected, and settled into a routine of accepting the shocks of growing up. After marrying Nils Jardine, she worked as a clerk-typist for the local hospital and quietly added to her duties until she became indispensable to the administrator, who recognized her growing abilities and rewarded her growth and efficiency.

Her longer hours put strains on the marriage with Nils who expected more attention from a loving wife. Shirley usually found time for Jenni but the last few years had been abnormally trying as she attempted to balance career, wifely and motherly duties.

As part of her coming of age at work, the administrator enrolled Shirley in the hospital's training program conducted by Dr. Tom Geiselman, an affable and tireless authority on medical management. He introduced Shirley and her classmates to cycles.

"People, their environment, and even the Universe all function in regular up and down cycles," Dr. Geiselman explained in answer to a question about why there seemed to be so much conflict in the world of work. *"The idea is to understand the rhythm and harmony and get into the flow of it,"* he urged the group.

He pointed out that Nature shows herself to be highly regulated in four seasons, the calendar as laid out by the Gregorian monks has twelve separate segments, and the world seems to operate in nine and thirty year epochs, repeating itself on an almost certified routine. What's important about this, the good doctor said, is that knowledge is power. *"Successful people use their intuition and rationality in a give-and-take process, exercising their whole brain to capitalize on situations. Hunches, or intuition, can be developed just as effectively as the more frequently used logic and linear thinking,"* he pointed out.

"Biorhythms, for example, tell us when we have the best of our physical, mental, and emotional energy going for us. That's when to throw yourself into life with gusto. That's not to say we shouldn't on other days, but the body does need time to rest and regenerate—on those days, perhaps it's better to plan or critique," he said, clarifying, in response to the questioning looks on some faces. When you know you're own up and down cycle, you're less apt to succumb to pressures to try and get high.

The idea of getting into your own rhythm makes sense and can be seen in those drug-free individuals, who schedule activities with regard for optimum use of their time and talents. *"I'm a morning person,"* you've heard someone say, or someone seems to catch fire later in the day and can stay up to all hours performing to the highest expectations. Where possible, it's a good idea to go with your natural instincts. You'll feel better and do better.

Unfortunately, we can't always do that—most places where we work don't consider your rhythm when utilizing you—so we adapt to their timeclock. Both suffer a productivity loss as a result. It would be best to work out a schedule where all employees could be in tune.

IN GOD WE TRUST

Further exploration into Shirley's nature indicated a strong spiritual link. She believed in God although she didn't belong to any special denomination. Her early exposure to religion had been ecumenical and nothing took firm hold of her, yet her instinctive reaction to a Supreme Power was undeniable. She prayed in her own way—a conversational talk with a Heavenly Father—and raised Jenni the same way. When she read more about what her numbers meant, she nodded in agreement.

Her lessons took her to some outside reading. One book, which she found fascinating, was written by Manly Hall. *Self Unfoldment* helped her understand that she needed a philosophy of life to reach her potential. Philosophy was not exclusively reserved for the scholars, the rich, nor the intellectual. Everyone needed a path to follow, a way of being. Hall helped Shirley see her instinctive link with the Universe. Through other insights and learning, she developed as a whole person and it was in this opening stage that Jenni confided in her.

When Shirley walked along her favorite pond nowadays, she began to notice more about how the ecology of life worked for the fish and small animals. This new realization combined with what she was learning from Dr. Geiselman gave Shirley a newfound confidence, especially where Jenni was concerned. She had grave doubts about Nils—she didn't seem to get through to him, despite a variety of approaches. Tenderness didn't work. Quietly abiding his misbehavior didn't work. Talking didn't help at all. Neither, it seemed, did conjugal love.

But where Jenni was concerned, it was good fortune that Shirley—mother and career prospect—was in a growth cycle. Had she not been, Jenni would have resorted to others for comfort and solace. And as she recounts, it would have been dangerous.

While the first years of life are critical in forming who we are and will be, most of that imprinting is at other than conscious levels. Jenni and her counterparts—whether in last grades of grammar school or junior high—experienced growth in so many different areas of their lives, faster and more intensely than they had or ever will. Adolescence is a time of conscious imprinting. Our juices are flowing, our feelings are wig-wagging and our efforts to be accepted are often misread, and rejected.

Never will our senses be so alert and open. It's a time of being alive and being scared to death of it all. This top of the mountain, bottom of the valley phase of development also carries a life threatening risk. More teens die of accidents than any other cause. Drinking/driving, drownings, guns, drugs, and the like goes with the adolescent lifestyle of "trying anything, any dare." Underlying it all is a huge cavernous need to be liked.

Jenni's new relationship with her mother came at a propitious time for her. When most daughters begin a rebellious stage of their growth and often turn away from parental guidance, Jenni shared her new, unbridled energy with a mother who was experiencing similar doubts and changes—a period of breaking out of an old rut and attempting to establish new ways of living.

Being able to talk about the wackiness of it all, on a person to person level, created a new and symbiotic relationship, which few parents and children achieve. Their experience went against a culture that provided strict roles for each. Parents are supposed to be in charge and children are expected to follow the examples of their elders. Maybe it's a good thing they do rebel and attempt to shake off some of the conformity with which society cloaks them.

While Shirley's breaking out was not as emotionally hill-and-valley as Jenni's, it was as far-reaching and wide. It proved, too, that adults can adapt from a lifetime of imprinting. But the serendipitous merging of mother and daughter periods of growth, saved at least one life. While it didn't save a faltering marriage, Jenni became the recipient of new ways of seeing things—just in time.

THERE, BUT FOR THE GRACE OF GOD

Jenni's best friend and confidant, Tina, found herself in a deep pit of despair after an awkward and humiliating row with her new boyfriend, a standout on the junior varsity football team. While she couldn't recall just what started the fuss, she knew that it ended horribly—or so she felt. Another acquaintance offered help—a chemical substance. One trip led to another and Tina soon found herself to be a teenage junkie.

Tina kept in touch with Jenni during this time, but didn't tell her about the drugs until she had become addicted. Adolescents often act in bizarre and uncertain ways, so it was not overly conspicuous that Tina was on drugs. Her mood swings had always been characteristic of her behavior. When she suggested Jenni try some, the problem became apparent.

"You've got to be kidding, Tina," Jenni fumed. *"I've got enough on my mind without worrying about how this stuff is going to react on my body. How long have you been doing this crap?"*

"Don't be a holier-than-thou, Sweet Pants. Just because you've become a Momma's Girl doesn't put you on a pedestal. I get enough of that at home without listening to you. Forget I asked. You can go home and stuff it," Tina said, walking away. A week later she was dead of an overdose. She was alone when it happened. A national statistic at age 14.

Jenni did say *"No"* as the advertisements on television prompted but she had plenty of help at home and in school. Before Jenni and her mother discovered their new potential together, Ruth Stock played a pivotal role in the teen's development. Ruth was a teacher's teacher, and a pupil's teacher. Not the spinster school marm by any stretch of the imagination, Ruth lived her own life as well as dedicating the prescribed time and then some to education.

"It's often difficult to remember that it's education you're really in, once the bell rings," Ruth explained how the schoolroom is the front line in the war on drugs. *"A teacher has many constituents to serve all at the same time—youngsters*

with potential, administrators with pet projects, school boards with pet concepts, a community with great expectations, other teachers with varied interests, and of course a personal home life. The most exciting to me is the classroom, even though I'm now a vice principal and part of the administration, I still find time to spend with the kids who are sprouting wings."

Pressures are on the school system right now. In many cases the whipping boy of a society caught unawares by the scope of the drug problem, schools take the brunt of the blame. President Reagan said it's an education problem to be solved. So did his wife, Nancy. The Congress of U.S. expressed similar sentiments. School officials admit it's in their jurisdiction. Then the consensus falls apart. When it comes to how to educate young people to resist the lure of alcohol and drugs, the leadership of a nation splinters into many pieces.

FROM A TEACHER'S POINT OF VIEW

Ruth Stock, though, knows what works. She doesn't have a magic wand or a fancy formula—it's just spitting on your hands and doing the hard work that has to be done. It's taking the time to learn about the medical aspects of addiction, the tell-tale signs of users and abusers, and doing what it takes to involve more parents and members of the community to help kids as they grow up.

"I'd say the biggest lesson to be learned is how to listen and that goes for the kids as well as adults. Teachers often find it hard to listen to individuals in a class. Those who do stay youthful and effective. Those who don't fall into terrible patterns of stuffiness and incompetence. A good teacher can and also should be a good friend," she said, offering a small blue-print for success.

A paradox of sorts is that teens seem to be torn between living up to what's in their genetic schematic and to changing it. Maybe that's what makes for so much excitement during these years. Some even seem to want it all—being both what was predetermined and what they fantasize about. It distills itself, in the long run, in whether they find unconditional love.

As Ruth Stock pointed out, a thoughtful and empathetic teacher kindles warmth and appreciation for youthful exuberance, reducing the anxiety that floods that very being. But it seldom becomes as deep as love can be.

Good friends can replace the family, at least for a portion of these tempestuous years. Yet even the most intimate of these relationships often fall short of unconditional love. Too many times, these friendships are eventually competitive at the base. The competitive nature of adolescence keeps peer relations above the truest of love. Peer pressure, on the other hand, provokes follow-me behavior, which can be overcome with full and committed love.

Normally in the family is where the true love can blossom and be the most heartfelt. Shirley and Jenni developed it there. And together they nurtured it to a higher and more satisfying level. They discovered what many in America are discovering—you can get high without drugs. They found out—like the bumper stickers say, "The It, of course, is Love."

PUT A LITTLE LOVE IN YOUR LIFE

The skeptics and the social critics label religious beliefs with an umbrella indictment. It goes something like, "God helps those who help themselves." Like many arguments against faith and belief, it is true. The skeptics say it in a snide and deprecating manner, however.

The believers realize that God, the Supreme Being, Divinity, Universal Truth, and similar designations for the Creator does not provide a step-by-step rote diagram for Love. Strong effort is needed to get there. Not always serious, not often joyful, the journey is an up and down one with many detours and sidetracks. Sometimes it begins at home, sometimes in church; most often it starts with self-realization. This understanding is true throughout the world's foremost religions, where more concepts are in common than practices are in conflict.

Statistically, the major religions account for more than two thirds of the world's nearly 5 billion inhabitants. About 30% are

Christians, 14% are followers of Mohammed, 12% are Hindu; 12% follow a number of Chinese folk beliefs; 5% are Buddhists; 2% are Shinto, and Jews account for less than 1%. Some people lay no claim to any organized beliefs and the rest are agnostics and atheists.

A comparison of historical precedents and current status brings these various religious beliefs into clearer focus. First, all generally agree that it's their role to help man and woman search for a path to salvation. They may call it differently, yet it boils down to finding that special gift inside of each of us that will enable us to be more than we thought possible.

To some this gift means answering the question, "Who Am I?" Christians answer it by explaining their relationship to Jesus. They also depict the goal of salvation as the purpose for people who are exposed to the trials of a lifetime on earth. Temptation such as drugs are a part of the Christian process. Crusaders, in search of salvation, a path toward a reunion with the Creator, win some of the battles and lose some. In the end, those who are Christians turn away from temptation and repent for having strayed.

Jews reply with a belief that you become one with God. They also identify the crusade as a search for justice—the balancing of the scales for people caught in the predicament of life.

Oriental religions suggest it's harmony with Universal nature. Use of drugs, for example, goes beyond a natural way of life and is counter to their belief. They use herbs as a way to keep themselves healthy and a strategy to return to equilibrium.

Buddhists, Christians, Jews, and others all talk of learning lessons while here on earth. They produce principles and guidelines for their followers to learn. Buddhists have the notion that suffering, excessive desire, renunciation of desire and following an eight step action outline are the significant features of life on earth. Hindus believe that you are born and die again and again until you learn the qualities that allow you to merge with God.

Rev. Robert E. Conover of the Calvary Presbyterian Church in San Francisco puts it this way: *"Christians know that God* takes them seriously—He offered his Son to clear the way for them to enter Heaven. Jesus, during his stay on earth, was tempted by the same things as other humans. He showed that these temptations were not always easy to shrug off, sinning was inevitable for most, but that a return to good standing—harmony, equilibrium, and balanced scales—was always possible. The parable of the prodigal Son remains viable today."

While each offers its congregation different rules, procedures, and guidelines, written and verbal, they each speak clearly of the basic virtues of truth, beauty, and goodness. They each speak of a spiritual philosophy as essential to understanding the answer to the question "Who Am I?" They all generally agree that life is cyclical—a natural give-and-take series of opportunities to learn who you are.

The idea of "rebirth or a return to the Original Force" seems common throughout the world and makes a statement to those seeking to crush out the drug menace today. Children will continue to experience as much of the world as they can in an effort to grow up. They will fall victims of serious temptations unless given as many tools as society can muster. One of the tools an impatient adolescent can learn as soon as possible is a philosophical one--an operating set of guidelines that includes a differentiation of right and wrong, a belief system built around the core values of their parents and a practical way of applying both.

The sooner children learn about Nature's cycles, the sooner they'll learn about their own cyclical nature. They'll see that you don't win them all, but that you can increase your winning percentage by being more aware of what's going on around you and how to adapt to trial, pain, suffering, and misfortune. Through a thoughtless rejection by a schoolmate, they can grow to understand that people have good days and bad ones. Knowing the whims of Nature can be useful in knowing what to expect, or knowing not to expect too much or too little. Expectations are often the criminal element of the young mind.

WE'VE GOT YOUR NUMBER

One approved way to learn more about your cycles and the natural inclinations of others is through numerology. Numbers play an important part of all our lives, and numerology, although obscured under a basket of the offbeat and occult for years, is a metaphysical science from which we all can learn and benefit. Gail Sheehy's "Passages" was one popular book based on a predictable pattern of age cycles. Any student of higher mathematics can quote bible and verse on what Pythagoras and his study of numbers meant to early civilization and ours today. Each number has a cycle, or vibration, of its own. This intimation is especially intriguing to young minds, which grasp the one-through-nine scheme of things quickly and clearly, once they get the hang of it.

Shirley Jardine and her daughter Jenni got in touch with each other partly through numbers. She learned that her name and birthdate provided her with a set of numbers, which can be used to interpret the ups and downs of her co-existence with Nature. Shirley was born on March 3, 1943 and in numerologic terms she had a life's purpose number of 5. According to the numbers people this means she was destined to experience life's opportunities thoroughly, rather than superficially.

To find out more what this meant to her, Shirley talked with some authorities on the subject. Joe Ivory, an accountant and credit manager with a major San Francisco paper company, and Georgia Stathis, a Chicagoan with masters in business administration, helped Shirley understand what hints and clues her numbers could give her. She also learned more about cycles. Joe and Georgia believe in the Pythagorean theory that birth numbers come equipped with patterns and cycles. Whether you believe in the numerologic explanations as Georgia and Joe do, it provides for some interesting and plausible focus of thinking. It did for Shirley.

She discovered that the universe follows nine-year cycles and so does she. The first year is for planting; the second for collecting sun and energy; the third for cultivating; the fourth for weeding out; the fifth for allowing growth; the sixth for clearing out; the seventh for deepening roots; eight for harvesting; nine for renewal. If you look at annual cycles as tides you'll see that one, three, and five are in, while two, four and six are out. Seven is way out and eight has brought the ship close to you. The ninth year is an inner-outer with both action and patience being apparent.

Because Shirley's yearly progression is the same as the universe—her One Year is the universal One—it was easy for her to determine some insights into her ins and outs. For instance, when she decided to leave Nils (an act of courage because of her spiritual convictions for strong family ties), she was in a four-year—a time to correct errors of the past. On the universal level, the four-year suggests a clearing away of the old and unworkable to make room for new growth.

For some, a four-year is a time for reconstruction and reorganization—a slimming down, a modernization. For others, it simply means getting down to basics, making work what you have available—putting the resources together in the most productive fashion, a systems approach.

This may seem in contradiction to some religious doctrine; Catholics, especially, hold a strong, dogmatic cincture about divorce. Shirley, however, did not divorce Nils—she separated herself from a man who repeatedly broke his word about drinking and became too much for her at this stage of her development.

Her action put the ball in Nils court. She could no longer live to her potential with this alcoholism albatross around her neck. No matter how she tried to help him and disengage herself, she couldn't shake it loose. Shirley believed that he would have to face up to himself before a reconciliation would be possible.

TWO HEADS ARE BETTER THAN ONE

Then Shirley discovered even more potential in the alliance of mother and daughter, who together might be able to provide a backdrop against which Nils could come to grips with his temptations. While this arrangement is supported by Alcoholics Anonymous and AlaNon, the organization for families of alcoholics, her discovery took on a more lyrical connotation. it seems that mother and daughter may have been destined to help Nils with his trouble.

Jenni Jardine was born Jenni Lynn Jardine on August 3, 1963. For numerologists, her birthdate meant she has a life purpose or destiny of a 3—someone who mixes well the aggressive aspects of male energy with the intuitive aspects of the feminine; a balance that usually results in creativity and self-expression. Numerologists also tell us her growth and development during her first 28 years will be influenced by a number 5—she will be challenged by the traits and characteristics of this number, hinting at some intolerance or prejudice. In other words, she must learn to overcome intolerance or bias to certain people and events.

Shirley, remember, had a number 5 life number. She also has a 5 as a challenge from age 29 to 56, and a 5 as an ongoing challenge—she would constantly have to keep from being too cavalier with life, too flighty. How Georgia and Joe explained this to her is that she needed to persevere in situations that didn't seem easy to her.

Nils was born on June 2, 1941. His life number is a 5. What this meant was that Shirley, at age 44, was smack in the middle of a 5 challenge, Nils. Jenni, too, had the same challenge.

When they listened to this being spelled, Jenni and Shirley Jardine were still. When it sank in, they looked at each other and made an unspoken commitment. They would make a dynamic duo, first for themselves and second for building a forum where Nils could work out his troubles without disrupting their growth. They could have come to this conclusion without the numerology. That's what more scientific types would say. The facts, though, speak for themselves. The numbers gave them some insight into their own growth potential and a person on which it could serve a noble and useful purpose—their father and husband, respectively. Figure 2.1 features an easy-to-use numerologic index for computing your own chart.

Nils became a challenge for the women in the best sense of the word. He became their life project. Nils became an integral

NUMEROLOGY INSTRUCTIONS

To determine your Personal Year, tally the birth month and day with the Universal Year. You get the Universal Year by adding the digits of the current year. For example, 1987 adds to a 7: 1 + 9 + 8 + 7 = 25 and the digits of 25 are 2 and 5 which when added equals 7.

Some one born on March 17 would have a 9 Personal year. March is a 3, added to 17 equals 20. Since 1987 is a 7, you add 20 and 7, getting 27, 2 + 7 = 9. In 1986, that person was going through an 8 year. In 1988, he or she experienced a 1 year.

To determine your Life's Lesson or Destiny, you work with your birth day, month, and year, adding up that total. Someone born on July 4, 1950 would have a Destiny of 8.

July is the seventh month, 7, add 4, getting 11 and the 15 from the year (1 + 9 + 5 + 0 = 15) and the total is 26 or 2 + 6 = 8.

If you were born on January 8, 1931, you'd have a destiny of a 5. 1 + 8 + 1 + 9 + 3 + 1 = 23, 2 + 3 = 5.

The bibliography contains names of resources for more information on numerology, astrology, and metaphysics.

Figure 2.1. Numerology instructions for determining your personal year.

part of the self-help process. This happened coincidentally because of what his boss saw happening both on the job and at home. What goes around, comes around. What happens at work tends to influence life on the ranch as well, and vice versa.

THE WORLD OF WORK
OFFERS EMPLOYEE ASSISTANCE

Since the calamitous rise in employee health care and related benefits, costs have gone unchecked over the past 14 years. Many of America's corporations and other major employers have undertaken serious measures to relieve this growing economic pressure. The U.S. Department of Commerce reported that American corporations spent more that $191 billion in 1986 to cover bills for doctors, hospitals, insurance premiums, and medical benefits. Ironically, this nearly matched the $201 billion in profit the same companies earned that year.

To deal with this queasy equation some are resorting to Health Maintenance Organizations (HMOs) which offer prevention as well as medical services for a set fee per employee per billing period. Others have formed consortiums called Preferred Provider Organizations (PPOs) to utilize doctors and hospitals at preset rates to regulate as much as possible the benefits outlay. Despite their best efforts, the costs continue a steady and seemingly irreversible climb.

Some of the more enlightened companies are trying a variety of employee-centered programs aimed at

1. lowering the prices at the point of delivery through competitive practices, volume purchasing (HMOs and PPOs) and putting together new and unique benefit configurations; and

2. lowering the amount of services used by employees without precluding access to necessary care.

The latter effort includes wellness programs, employee assistance plans, and assorted health-seeking and fitness ideas. In this constructive web is where Nils found himself caught. Nils' boss had become part of a corporate lifestyles program and as such noticed the aberrant behavior of several of his work unit. Ben Giles had been a considerate, yet forceful and aggressive manager. Before his training in the lifestyles program, Ben would not have said much to Nils even if he had noticed a turn in his performance. Oh, he may have cajoled him a little or taken him out to lunch and hinted at his misgivings, but he wouldn't have taken any bold steps to confront the issue. Those kinds of personal relations were best left to the experts, Ben believed. Getting product out was his job.

Today, things are different. Companies such as New York Telephone, Kimberly Clark, Control Data, IBM, and others have pioneered the concept that a healthy employee is a productive one. The research shows they go hand in hand. Chief executives and financial officers are taking note of it. This has led the way to hundreds of organizations, large and small, public and private, to see economic as well as human benefits from taking a more personal regard for all employees, starting as usual with management types.

Ben Giles was one of the first managers to be trained in a new health and productivity system. He was not a likely candidate—Ben was a natural skeptic. He was set in his ways and not apt to change his thinking or behavior unless thoroughly convinced it was worth it. After looking at the program and taking part in the preliminary orientation, Ben became intrigued and soon became one of its leading exponents.

As such he became aware of and skilled in nutrition, relaxation, exercise, and support systems on one side and project management on the other. He became fascinated with the concept and practice of turning excessive stress into useful and healthy energy. Before learning this system he had been demonstrative but not confrontive. He changed his behavior—slowly at the start and gradually he saw that trouble was really energy going the wrong way. Through confrontation, he could redirect and channel energy towards creative solutions.

Like Shirley Jardine, and without benefit of knowing she was learning similar skills, he perked up considerably at the notion of cycles. As an electrical engineering major with an economics minor in college, he found he could relate easily to peaks and valleys of human behavior. It reminded him a little of theories on wave guides and capital growth. They used a cyclical approach.

Old friends and co-workers of Ben were surprised of a sort when Ben not only confronted the situation with Nils but that he had taken the time to plan a sophisticated strategy for how to get at the heart of Nils alcoholism. The company had set specific goals for productivity and employee benefits cost containment and control. Ben became an intern in the new health and productivity program.

CONNECTING PERSONAL ISSUES TO CORPORATE AND NATIONAL INTERESTS

Senator John McCain, Republican from Arizona and replacement for the retiring Barry Goldwater, joined the Commerce committee with an agenda designed to spark interest in corporate productivity as a way to compete more effectively with companies overseas, especially those on the Pacific Rim and in Europe. Without a national industrial policy, according to congressional critics, this country is handicapped in its dealings with foreign competitors who have the advantages of lower wage rates, vested government and corporate protection, and sub rosa ethical practices.

Senator McCain, and others, believes American industry has much more untapped potential than it recognizes. On the other side of the aisle and in the other house, Representative Richard Gephart, Democrat from Missouri, believes that the American worker, too, has been short-shrifted. Congressman Gephart believes Americans can be just as quality and cost-conscious as foreign workers—properly motivated. He points to the Fremont, California plant where General Motors and Toyota jointly produce cars with fewer rejects, higher output, and lower costs than GM did when it owned and operated the plant without Japanese management methods.

McCain and Gephart are onto something. The key is motivation. Not the usual carrot- and-stick approach, but inner motivation—the kind that lasts during the tough times. The product of real motivation is health and productivity. The icing on the cake is that it's also a part of prevention plan for addiction.

FROM THE HALLOWED HALLS
OF CORPORATE AMERICAN

More and more corporations are coming to understand that a healthy employee is a productive one. It used to be that the human relations movement of the 1950s and lasting into the 1980s that happiness and satisfaction were believed to be what created productivity. This may be partially true but not comprehensive enough to be institutionalized. The partial truth has led many people and their employers to do some strange things in the way of motivation; some worked to a certain extent, none for any length of time.

For instance, motivational theorists believe that the employee's family plays an important part in his or her satisfaction. To reach that trigger, they put company picnics in the employee benefits package. There is not one shred of evidence that the annual picnic does one bit of good, indirectly or directly to the balance between the employee and subsequent performance. The link between a concern for the employee, the family, and productivity is remote if in fact real.

While the price may be small to pay, the relative worth of the picnic would be better served in a more direct and constructive fashion. Say a picnic costs the company $30,000 a year. In ten years, a sum of $300,000 could have been better invested in a private park or lodge that families could use when they scheduled it to conduct family picnics and outings of more lasting and less dubious quality.

The same can be said for the current fad of employee assistance, wellness, and similar programs aimed at restoring harmony in familial situations. Some of these plans and actions do serve a purpose, for a few. The cost effectiveness, however, of most miss the original intent. Not enough and often not the right people take advantage of them. The corporate gym and park may look inviting, but the alcoholic, drug abuser, and obese rarely participate on a regular and coordinated schedule.

Robert Rosen, editor of Corporate Commentary, evaluates a number of health care programs for companies and wistfully says the value of such efforts are at best questionable. "When companies begin to manage their people differently, they'll show signs of better health and increased productivity." By differently, Rosen means showing genuine concern and thoughtful planning, not allowing work to be done in a chaotic, stressful, and reactive environment.

Erich Fromm has written extensively about man's need to overcome an innate isolation. Worksites, even with a constant din of people chattering and machines whirring, can be lonely. Psychologist Fromm suggested that we begin educating people at an early age, childhood and adolescence, to learn how to be alone without being lonely.

Once the isolation fear has been eliminated, or at least curbed to a survival coping level, people will be able to deal more effectively with their down cycle. The downer is certain to come in even the most adaptive of people. We all rip off a button at an inopportune time, spill a drink or forget an important date or meeting—these are minor insults to our character. We don't need to lie on the psychiatrist's couch for these embarrassments. We need to understand that some mistakes are not fatal—we all are flawed.

The psychiatrist has a role to play, a reconstructive one usually, but not in these menial venues. We can handle one, two, or more of these at a time, if we've had the basic training early on in life. We can even do quite well despite childhood deprivation of this training.

ON A MORE PERSONAL LEVEL

What's important is to know your own pattern of ups and downs. When they start. What triggers they. What to do about them. If cycles are a personal system of yours, the more you know about the particulars, the better off you'll be.

Most people have a friend that's an accident going somewhere to happen. We call these friends klutzy, clumsy, fumblefingers, or just plain out of it. They have a built-in magnet for trouble. At the same time, they resist total destruction with equal dexterity. They may get hurt, but never maimed. They always have a band-aid on their body; their closets are filled with torn garments; their cars look like they just came from target practice. The cycle, in their case, is frequency-centered, not amplitudinal. The degree of injury, embarrassment, or luck is constant, although limited in scope.

On the other hand, we all have experienced more serious cases of the death wish. This is the individual who, on command, will self-destruct just when victory or completion of a task or assignment is at hand. They possess all the skills, charm, and fortitude to win against all odds, except to finish the race. The boss and spouse are over for dinner: the night is perfect, the meal sumptuous, the stories funny, and, at the door saying goodnight, they commit a policy indiscretion—they mention a raise or promotion or like that.

Instead of feeling themselves being pulled into the abyss, they rush headlong into the death plunge. Despite countless experiences of similar events, they lose control of their equilibrium and dive for the bottom. They pump their limbs feverishly to hasten the demise. They lock-step the process with an engineering precision. Later, they recall the event with sad and forlorn looks of dismay. *"I saw it coming, but couldn't get out of the way."*

Drug abusers say that a lot.

They miss all the symptoms of their down cycle. They get steadily down on themselves until, in their way of thinking, it's time to get high—through chemicals. Rather than being alert to the trend, they react only when the opportunity for recovery has passed. A big part of the problem is not knowing your choices.

Psychologist Erich Fromm noted that "man cannot live without some sort of cooperation with others." The quality of the cooperation gives substance to the existence. It also can be said that man and woman cannot live without choices to determine the quality of their lives.

From childhood on, we've been told to put limits on ourselves: don't play in the street; don't touch the stove; don't write on the walls; don't do this or that. While the injunctions are generally useful and enable us to avoid calamity, the insistence of negative dos and don'ts tend to dominate our early, dependent days. In time, what seems to many of us to be our only choices of behaviors are amongst a set of restrictions.

While parents and elders meant us no harm, in fact were attempting to keep us alive to live another day, they did us another type of harm—they limited our perspective on choices. If we failed to heed the warnings from elders, we'd likely experience pain, cause some material damage to our surroundings or at least run out the string of patience they had in trying to bring us up.

But this may have happened at a great cost. This mindless acceptance of negative injunctions may have dampened our ability to grow from experience. We may have stifled a more full use of learning how to discriminate one action from another. We may have chilled a chance for quicker and more lasting independence or, to put it another way, the ability to select for ourselves.

That's not to say we don't need care and attention during our early, formative years. We certainly do. But a better way does exit than impose such a preponderance of negativism.

A GIFT TO BE NURTURED

Take the exceptional child for example. Every school teacher in the world is pleased to identify that child who soaks up teaching like a sponge, asks the pertinent question, and brings joy to an otherwise drab although noisy classroom. The trouble is that today's schools, with a few notable exceptions, are not set up to deal with the uncommon child.

The teacher is torn between encouraging independence of thinking and action and the need to keep order and conformity in the class. The choice, in most of these cases, unfortunately, is made for the rest of the class. Unless the guardians of the gifted child have the where-withall for private school or special classes, the child does not receive the attention necessary to bring out the best of the early gifts.

So society, too, has been limited in its choices. Parents are, teachers are and we pass this onto our children. This is not the legacy many of us had in mind when we set out to provide more for our offspring than we had ourselves.

Fromm pointed out that we either adapt to conditions statically or dynamically, which is to say that we either change our behavior without changing our character, static, or we incorporate the change so that the entire character structure is impacted. Immigrants coming to America adapt statically when they put aside chop sticks and use forks and knives or learn English as a second language. A dynamic adaptation can be seen when the newcomer accepts new neighbors, quickly learns to trust them and becomes assimilated into the new society with little or no reservation.

On the down side of dynamic adaptation is when a child, for instance, submits to commands from a parent to be a "good" boy or girl, but harbors a resentment. The child is too dependent on the parent to rebel, but this resentment, when repressed, can develop into an intense hostility. This is the rule today rather than the exception because of the negative injunctions issued in early childhood.

The child learns limited choices. In the above case, he or she is too weak or dependent to voice objections to the stronger more dominant adult. Should the child voice objections—attempt to enter into a dialogue with the adult—they are usually punished, starting a whole line of more limiting treatment, such as "go to your room," to spankings, to visits to the psychologist.

In a perfect world, parents will be granted more patience and skill in helping children develop their natural abilities. In the meantime, parents will be hassled by seeming irrational behaviors and react in kind. While some children harbor the unconscious grudge against the one parent, many simply transfer it to the world in general. Their anxieties toward authority figures throughout early childhood may lead to deeper submission of true feelings and finally wind up with a vague but persistent defiance that shows up from time to time.

Neurosis is an example of dynamic adaptation. Some of us are more or less neurotic over some aspect of human life. None of us escape the dilemma of working with others without conflict.

Not having the full set of skills to function smoothly day in and day out without getting dinged here and there is our lot.

A huge part of the problem lies in the suppressed emotional energy that began when we were young, weak, dependent and growing up. We have learned to limit, so we do so in reaction to all external stimuli.

Not all of our limitations are the same. Some of our choices to what life offers are flexible, especially in adolescence when our needs are being more visibly defined. The path we choose is open. We can go right, left, or straight ahead. Though we are generally governed by what our parents direct us to, we may react differently if the hostility is great enough or deep enough.

In other cases, we are more rigid. We don't have an option to eat or not eat, to sleep or not sleep. We accept a certain number of needs and adapt only to the extent of how much we eat in a given set of circumstances or how long we sleep.

In the case of getting started on drugs or booze, we are likely to make our choices based on current information about what it means to us, not so much what it means to our injunctors. That is to say, we are likely not to rebel against parents asking us not to, unless we are in a state of mind to recall our hostility against them. It also means that we need to know if it's harmful or not.

Then too, peer pressure comes into play as the third part of the decision-making process. First, we need to know what it means to us; second, what authorities say about it, and third, does it constitute a threat to our immediate circle of friends. If the first and second inputs cancel themselves out—we know it's dangerous to use them but we're deeply angry with Mom or Dad—we're likely to go along with the crowd. That's a Good News, Bad News catch. It's good that we go along with consensus, bad if they are into misbehaving or into experimenting.

SUMMARY

Growing up is a matter of making the best choices possible in a given set of circumstances. The more these choices follow a natural inclination, the more likely they are to be good for us.

Most people respect Nature and can learn from the ecology around them, provided some guidance is offered early and without negative influences. The ability to love is instinctive and can be nurtured through example and experience. The home is the best place for love to be unfolded.

Schools are changing and can be a force for proper character development of young people. Parents, teachers and children can work together, if parents and teachers give it a chance.

Adults can correct some of their early childhood mistakes later on—it's difficult but worth the effort.

Saying "No" is a behavioral expression that needs to be rooted in healthy soil and cared for by thoughtful gardeners. It's not enough to lip sync words without feelings of love and affection.

Chapter **3**

CHECK UNDER THE HOOD, PLEASE

People noticed that Tommy Ward looked taller than most ninth-graders—his jeans didn't touch his shoes and his sleeves barely reached his wrists, no matter how well they fit when just new. Lanky is what they called him. His growth spurt between 14 and 15 years caused a social as well as physical phenomenon. Being looked up to became an early part of Tommy's outlook on life. He didn't particularly welcome nor disdain it—it just was.

Besides the offhand jokes about never being able to keep him in clothes long enough to wear them out, his mother and father liked the idea that he seemed to have **"command"** presence. Tommy's father knew that tall people tended to be more respected, earned more money and in general made out better in life's material offerings.

Tommy eventually did take note that others tended to follow his lead more this year than last, and while this didn't dissuade him from doing what he wanted, he wondered about his leadership values. Every once in a while the pangs of conscious made their presence known to him at unusual times. Like once when one of his friends offered to share some marijuana with five of the guys after school. The other three looked to see what Tommy would do before they made their choice.

THE INNER MOTIVATION: BASIC VALUES

Distinguishing between what you need and what you want is one of the major learnings during adolescence. So much of early childhood is spent pleading, manipulating, and cajoling mom or dad to give you G.I. Joe, robots, gum and candy, and other "wants" that it comes as a shock that you don't really "need" these comforts and luxuries to function as a thoughtful and useful human being.

The distinction between needs and wants makes a lot of sense once it's understood. It provides a vehicle for realizing what motivates one to achieve life's purpose. For most American young people and many adults, however, the definition remains a blur. It's evident today in the conflict amongst the major powers of the world. They are propelled to compete militarily because of a lack of understanding each other's basic motives, or at least a mistrust of those motives. It's similar to kids in the school-yard arguing over what they "want" rather than "need."

Former Senator William Fulbright, Democrat from Arkansas, probably did more for foreign nations to understand their needs through a scholarship program he established in 1946 than all the so-called summit meetings put together. Nearly 50 nations have kept an elite corps of aspiring people enrolled in international relationship study during the forty years of the program and only now does there seem to be a payoff in the effort.

During a recent speech to the National Press Club in Washington, D.C., Senator William Fulbright smiled when asked why it took 40 years for the program to make inroads, saying, *"It takes that long for most people to get into powerful positions in their countries. People like the Prime Minister of Sweden, for instance, and other leading statesmen in other nations evolve into authority."* During this process, they see the commonality amongst people regardless of their national origins. Because of this exposure, they can appeal to fundamental beliefs across the political spectrum. The politics may differ widely; the people don't. His explanation was cogent, concise, and right on target.

What Fulbright was explaining, in part, is that a person's operating values system—most of which they learn early on and develop over time—does not make a national impression until they reach an elevated rank and status, which allows for a wide exposure. The same principle, however, holds true in lesser degrees for all of us. What we learn and retain of our character development at home and later in school is honed and refined throughout life.

Fulbright contends that education early on in understanding values is critical to world unity and peace. He points out that a people-to-people approach coupled with political negotiation will offer a more durable solution to world problems than a political and military combination.

Just as a Fulbright Fellowship allows a would-be diplomat to learn the techniques of international politics, the same scholar also learns the nature of the people in various countries and sees how similar their values are. In fact, a contention can be made that most all of the world's population may have the same core values wherever they acquire them. Prepostrous? Maybe not.

THE NATURE OF MOTIVATION

Since Freud brought psychology to popular useage, experts have pondered the question of what drives people to do what they do—what indeed does make Sammy run? Budd Shulberg wrote "What Makes Sammy Run?" during a time when America was getting used to psychology as a practical, not a theoretical science. People continue to search for answers to questions about behaviors.

From psychotherapy in its various formats through counselors in sundry coats—transactional analysis, family, career, marriage etc.—the public has been exposed to the causes and cures of neurotic behavior. What are the motives at work?

Conversationally, *neurosis can be described as "strange doings." The experts define it as out of normal*—and hardly anyone has been able to make other than a judgment call on norms.

When you go to court on a case such as the von Bulow murder trial, expert and credible witnesses line up on each side. The jury is out on nearly every verdict. Suffice it to say that some bartenders make good practical psychologists. Well, they should. Most neurotics, who drink, go to bars.

The biggest mystery to most Americans, however, remains that of motivation. Pop psychologists like Werner Ehrhard, through his est program, have become millionaires, easier than Freud, Adler, Jung and the truly respected practitioners in the field, talking to masses of people on the concept and practice of motivation. Every other channel on television talk shows features this expert or that on this fascinating and veiled subject.

Why do we do what we do?

"Money," that's what the materialistic say.

"No, it's not money. It's what money can get you," say another category of pundits.

"For me, it's family and the love within that motivates me," says the 33-year-old computer systems analyst.

"Hearing my boss and clients tell me how wonderful my project worked out," says the 41-year-old marketing professional.

"Making the pieces of a complicated work puzzle fit together is what turns me on," according to a 53-year-old government office supervisor.

"Getting the best out of a hopeless situation satisfies me," a 22-year-old university student responded.

More than 500 members of Entrepreneurs Alliance talked about motivation and it all boiled down to five, intertwined aspects of their different and changing lifestyles. They identified the core of motivation—a set of values that belongs to each of us—**competence, determination, teamwork, communications,** and **economics.**

Competence applies to both social and vocational skills. For the young person it's school grades that depict vocational abilities and the ability to get along with family, friends and others. ***Determination*** is the drive that makes for the best quality output of any effort—at home, work, or school. It's an intensity that matches the moment. ***Teamwork*** can be seen in a variety of ways. At home, it's sharing in the chores; at work, it's picking up the slack when one of the group is off ill or indisposed; socially, it's when you give blood, run a fund drive, or chauffeur the soccer team to its games. ***Communications*** is at its best when it's a two-way exchange of views, a dialogue. You communicate when you listen, too. ***Economics*** is complex as well. Not only is it money, the Bottom Line and cost consciousness, it can be psychic income—that feeling of reward you experience when the other four values were fully extended.

Whether young or old, blue or white collar, teacher or student, parent or child, the values are the same. The priority and intensity varies according to a number of factors, but the consensus is indisputable! What makes you do the good things in life are your values. When you do something contrary to your own belief system, it's usually because guilt or fear enmesh with the core values, turning them sour. They become the bad and ugly motivators.

Ask yourself what triggered your latest emotional outburst—anger, joy, sadness, happiness, grief—and you'll see a basic value that's been touched. Jill Rackley drove down the freeway, got cutoff by a rude driver, received an obscene gesture for her honk, and blew her cool. What happened? Two core values were in conflict, resulting in the penalty of a third motivator.

First, the other driver proved not to be ***competent,*** failed to ***communicate*** his intentions of changing lanes, and, second, when she honked the horn, he challenged her ***competence*** as a driver with a unprofessional ***communication.*** He paid the price—***economics***—when the highway patrol pulled him over for the lane violation.

Another illustration: Tom Bertken read the notice from school announcing his son's nomination to the Merit Honor

Society and warmly embraced the lad. Joy sprang from a combination of all the values. The youngster's obvious competence was coupled with a determination for quality. The family regarded good grades as especially important and communicated that in a variety of ways. Tom rewarded the top notch effort with a hefty increase in the weekly allowance—a win/win situation for parent and child.

Unfortunately, not everyone knows his or her value system as well as they might. Much of what passes for values are simply cliches or poor examples of these deep-seeded drives. The trials and tribulations in our lives can be traced to actions triggered by guilt or fear intrusions on our values.

Peters and Waterman in their spectacular business book success, *In Search of Excellence: Lessons from America's Best-Run Companies,* devoted an entire chapter to values and defined them, basically, in the same terms. Abraham Maslow described similar values as the rudiments for the self-actualized person—the successful, creative, and winning personality.

These and other researchers of what it takes to rise above the level of mediocrity that pervades alcohol and drug-influenced cultures also link **ongoing education**—learning everyday from life—as another ingredient in the success mixture.

Longshoreman and philosopher Eric Hofer wrote about "learning . . . as a source for discipline." The kind of discipline that adolescents, especially, need to cope with the fast changes of their lives. Hofer believed that the American society—based as it is on immigrants who had to adapt to new ways—is uniquely equipped to grow and mature in a creative and orderly fashion. In fact, he felt a responsibility of Americans was to do so. He called it the most essential ingredient in a good society.

Hofer's experience led him to believe that one primary function of a society is to allow opportunities for its people to become better. While this may seem pessimistic from one point of view, he was a realist who knew that the people of a non-learning society tended to follow and not lead. Followers find it difficult to change, and learning is all about change.

THE INTERCONNECTION OF
LEARNING AND CHANGE

Why it's so difficult to sell the idea of ongoing learning to a lot of people is inertia—the need for the pendulum to cease its swings and settle down comfortably in the middle. So many of us work hard to gain some status, a relative comfort level, and at some point want to stop and rest. Maybe we only intended the rest to be a temporary one, but once the momentum is lost—like the pendulum—we fall quietly.

Our history is one of birth, learn, work, retire, and die. Today some feel learning is a thread that continues from birth through the final moments and is not merely something you get and put on the mantel. A tendency also shifts to slow down once the retirement age approaches. It's not to say comfort and respite should be shunned. Nobel prize winner and octogenarian Linus Pauling feels that purpose of life is the thrill that makes it all worth while and keeps his cycle going. Without a vision of beauty, goodness and truth, the trial seems unworthy.

Franklin Buscher was a good example of someone who defied the quieting pendulum. He had good rhythm. His days and nights were consistent—it's as if he were programmed to concerted effort with regularly scheduled quiet times. The dull and monotonous routine work of a Navy yoeman could overcome even the most resolute and die-hearted. Not for Frank. He was well aware of his values and how to keep frustration at work at bay. His social life was similar.

Franklin bounced around on a sea of red tape. Orders from Washington sometimes countermanded the reality on base and the resulting confusion eventually led to inaction, an inertia of memorable proportions. People quit trying after a while. It just didn't seem worth the effort to change the tradition.

In fact, his favorite phrase was, *"...whatever's customary."* Then he'd go do it his way, which inevitably was quicker, more to the point, and surprisingly within the intent if not the letter of the law.

What turned out to be customary at this particular Navy installation was drug use—marijuana, amphetamines, uppers, downers and even a little heroin, a carryover from service in Viet Nam. Franklin was no prude, to be sure—he enjoyed fun and games as well as the next guy—but he put his foot down when it came to hard core.

He became a one-man education program against drugs. Like any good military strategist, Franklin did it by the book—his book, which was part Navy, part hometown values, and part seat-of-the-pants. He began by reading official regulations on substance abuse; he made judicious inquiries on policies and practices—you know, what was customary—and he discovered what media was available for education.

Before long, filmstrips, films, lectures, and discussions on the ills of drugs starting showing up in training sessions, the wardroom, the drill floor, and anywhere people tended to congregate. LSD no longer meant Lucy in the Sky with Diamonds.

The result was not officially recognized—in those days drug abuse was kept in the closet or brushed under the rug—so Franklin received no commendation for his effort. A few people knew and recognized his above and beyond the call of duty in a variety of ways. Some thanked him, others started to take this young and unusual American seriously—something he wanted very much.

One person can make a difference. For Franklin Buscher, an easier approach would have been to put in his time and let it go at that. He was not striking for any rate or stripes with his war on drugs. What he was doing was simply a matter of doing what was customary for him.

ONE MAN'S MEAT

Too many Americans, unfortunately, find change inordinately difficult to manage. American industrialists are some prime examples of resisting change. A country that once led the world in manufacturing proficiency now finds itself trailing other nations in steel production, losing ground in automobile share of market, and almost out of the textile arena entirely.

Electronics, semiconductors, radios, televisions, machine tools and others are areas where the U.S. has floundered and lost ground to the more flexible and attentive interests in Europe and the Orient, especially the Pacific Rim.

Going from the world's leading creditor to the leading debtor nation between 1975 to 1985 took some rigidity. Leaders, who were watching quarterly reports—a short-range view—were caught in this tunnel vision approach. Rather than risk changes in operations, equipment, materials, and management styles, some U.S. industries opted to remain firm in their direction. The rash of mergers, cutbacks, and shifts to offshore operations can be traced directly to inflexibility, flying in the face of opportunities crying for changes.

Granted, we are creatures of habit. Much of the time, though, the habit is nondescript. We go to work the same way, we bowl on Thursdays, we clean the garage every other Saturday, we become hospitable with our remarks.

Unlike the Franklin Buschers, we don't cultivate the welcome-change habit. This doesn't mean we have to reinvent the wheel for every circumstance. What is meant is that we should practice open mindedness and be tyranically suspicious of conformity.

Dr. Maxwell Maltz, who discovered the psycho cybernetics concept, believes you can develop a new habit in just 21 days of paying attention to it. His concept is that what gets on within the mind tends to get on the muscle. The good doctor tied together intellectual intentions with emotional practice. When you want it bad, or good enough, you'll get it and keep it.

His theory, which worked well with throwing darts, losing weight, and similar behavioral activities didn't do as well if those person undergoing change overlooked the energy of their value system. Dr. Maltz's locus of control concept connected mental and emotional energies, providing those persons could garner those elusive qualities. Too often they couldn't.

Behavior changes alone don't last. That's why the drug addict who knows in his or her own mind that quitting is the only solution to peace and quality of life, often can't keep with the promise because the feelings come and go—they usually go at the time push comes to shove. Emotional energy—feelings—is linked directly to one's values. In Figure 3.1 is illustrated how the energy works through the personality. Behavior and attitudes are energies of choice, while values aren't.

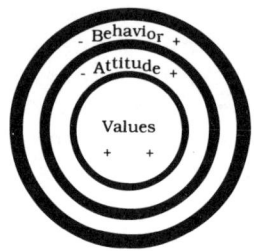

Figure 3.1 Illustration of how energy works through the personality.

Starting with a double positive, the core values, once understood, drive one to optimism, hope and achievement. When we come across a new situation in our lives, we have a choice—like the new experience, have doubts about it or dislike it. Somewhere along that continuum of options, we exercise our best judgment given some time to think about it. If we like it, and it comes through the screening test of our values, we'll tend to keep looking for situations similar to it.

If we didn't like it, or have some doubts about it, and that too doesn't fit our values, we'll probably disregard searching for others like it. Say we attend a soccer match for the first time. We may be with friends who like it, but it doesn't meet our expectations or value of a baseball game between the Yankees and Tigers, we'll probably not go out of our way to attend a second time. Our values influence our attitude, which in turn influences our behavior.

Contrarily, if we have a son or daughter who happens to go out for the junior high soccer team, makes it, becomes a standout player, our values have been tapped and the reverse comes about. We see the value of the game because it has taken on a more personal energy in our lives. We'll not only attend more games, but we may involve ourselves in learning the rules, the strategies, and even get into coaching some of the fundamentals. Like a Franklin Buscher, we'll exercise some simple behaviors with strong dedication and likely results because the energies go through attitudes clear down to values.

We'll accept the change of heart, from not having an opinion either way on soccer because now we are hooked—addicted in a positive sense to something new and something we wouldn't have given two cents for a year or so ago. Left alone, without influences, we would not exercise choice. **By dipping into the values bank, we come out with dividends.**

We have fun; we're learning and teaching some new skills; the family gains from our involvement as we have another chance to talk about life through sport; and hopefully the team gains from new energies exerted by a clear-cut set of values.

Dr. Maltz paved the way for a deeper understanding and commitment to habits. Now we can go even further with his concept. By helping young people learn their values, not like they learn the multiplication tables or fractions, we'll foster their natural creative energies, which usually go unattended or reversed because they take up too much time.

A pesty child can be trying. No doubt of that. Just look at the soaring cases of child abuse reported last year. The trouble is that the child is not to blame. They're built to express themselves in the manner best suited for their stage of development. Befuddled and confused parents create painful and criminal acts. They suffer emotional breakdowns and react savagely. These parents learned that behavior somewhere.

Bad or undesired behavior is correctable, though. We can unlearn any behavior. But we need to know the core driving motor mechanism. Each time we turn the child away, we miss an opportunity for clarifying their values for them—not an easy subject for them to learn. (A recent survey of drug abusing families indicated that among adult professionals only 15% knew what their values were and how they worked to motivate them—making a mockery of the "what you don't know, can't hurt you" idiom.)

HOME IS WHAT YOU MAKE IT

A jazz classic recorded in the 1950s by Billie Holliday—another tragic story of drug abuse—is titled "God Bless the Child." It tells about a family where the Momma has, Poppa has, and God bless the child that has his own. The meaning, of course, is that the child has picked up the skills for a joyful life. The skills for living can be acquired in only one perfect setting—the home.

Schools are extensions of the home and at best are, like art, imitators of life. The recent examinations of public schooling in this country by the Congress, the National Governors Conference, blue ribbon panels of all sorts agree that something drastic needs to be done to correct infirmities—a crippling condition that threatens the future of this country. (More on schools in later chapters.)

But schools can't be the scapegoat for substance abuse. People do drugs, not institutions. The most important of the formative years are spent at home even before schooling begins. The tape recorder of thoughts and feelings occur at birth and continue until the brain quits recording. The child learns critical skills at home. Not how to type, or keep accounts, or sell insurance, but the primary skills of give and take. These may be polished later in school and on the street, but basic training is in the living room and kitchen.

Developmental psychologist Erik Erikson researched the growth of children into adulthood and gave names and descriptions to each and descriptions to each level of advancement. He also worked with shell-shocked Army veterans, who became the first stress victims of a mighty nation at war. A third major work of his concentrated on why native Indian tribes in America rejected certain of the white man's cultural traits, choosing to remain in their own environment. This trilogy of Erikson's work serves as the foundation for this and one subsequent chapter.

Erikson discovered, and later confirmed by many including Abraham Maslow, that life's skills are products of early childhood. He identified eight of these skills and others have segmented the eight into twelve. Six are rational and six are intuitive.

The six rational skills tend to be logical, objective, and linear in nature, while the six intuitive skills are more spontaneous, subjective, and emotional. Lately, the skills have been associated with specific hemispheres of the brain—rational for left and intuitive for right—but nothing is quite so distinct, some overlap does occur.

In Figure 3.2 are listed the root need of the skill and a delineation of the skill.

Needs	Skills
Rational Skills	
Clarity	Job/Results Clarity
Achievement	Work Plans/Schedules
Industry	Problem Solving
Integrity	Indicators/Standards
Control	Feedback/Evaluation
Curiosity	Data Analysis
Intuitive Skills	
Trust	Data Collection
Intimacy	Know Needs of Others
Generativity	Close the Process
Self Identity	Know Self Needs
Autonomy	Keep Process Open
Initiative	Risk Taking

Figure 3.2. Rational and intuitive skills and related needs.

By looking at the roots of these skills, you get an idea of why they become so important in the growing up process. The first need most of us have is for **clarity.** Without a clear view of what's going on around us or where we intend to go, confusion reigns. Therapists, counselors, and friends are often called on to help something caught in a muddle. Clarity is the basis for the first of the rational, left-brained skills.

Every motivational scientist from Frederick Herzberg to McClellan to Werner Ehrhard and others in between cite the need to achieve as one of the foremost drives. **Achievement** is one of the major forces in a society, an organization, or an individual. It gives strength and purpose to life and binds even the most diverse elements or personalities. It's a common thread.

One of the first few words a child speaks is "why." Knowing how things work, **industry,** is the quest many follow all their lives. It keeps the midnight oils burning and provides other fuel for the problem solvers of life. One of the reasons it will remain so relevant is because of opportunity—problems to solve always will be present in a culture as adversarial as ours. It's a requisite for success or good health.

High on the list of any trait or characteristic for wholeness is **integrity.** A person's word is his/her bond which has long been the trait of quality, honesty, and virtue. Being true to yourself first and to others has been extolled from pulpits, repeated in relationships, and admired in every recorded civilization. Taking pride in your efforts and yourself keeps you distinct and separate from lower forms of animal life.

Since the universe has been one of the most studied wonders of our existence, its sense of order has been a factor to emulate—a driving force for its inhabitants. People want to know what's coming, no surprises, to be in charge of events and even themselves. **Control** is that need. It's a discipline of our relations and activities—the essence of cooperation for optimum results.

The fact that detective and mystery novels continue to outsell other fiction is no surprise. People are naturally curious.

Curiosity may have killed the cat, but it makes for human progress on a variety of levels. Our need to analyze and critique our experiences keeps us alert to new and exciting opportunities. Satchel Page may not have liked to look back for fear someone was gaining on him, but most of us want to know the lay of the land—we're insatiably curious.

These six needs are predominantly housed in the left side of the brain. They are associated with verbal, thinking, mathematical, and the hard sciences. The next six are more nonverbal, emotional, spatially related, and closer to the softer sciences.

When a baby is born and is held closely by the mother to her breast and fondled lovingly by the father, ***trust*** is nurtured in that infant. Without physical and emotional stroking, the child is said to suffer trust deprivation—a condition that prevents him or her from relating to the surrounding world in a close and healthy manner. This need, if not cultivated during the first year and continued throughout adolescence, causes serious problems—conflicts and poor choices for relationships.

Psychoanalyst Eric Berne described ***intimacy*** as a loving nature of people. He distinguished it from sexual love and noted that intimacy was the ability to get close to someone without losing yourself in the process. It's been described as being authentic, real with someone else—no games being played. It's a warm and fuzzy kind of need. A rare one in today's technologic society. One that remains insistent over the years and does not fade with so called maturity.

Generativity, according to Erikson, is a built-in need for procreation, a thoughtful view of what's best for the next generation. It can be seen practiced and fulfilled by people who work for clean air, clean water, drug-free schools, and the rest of ecology. They also keep their neighbors in mind when caring for their own yard and garden. Generativity is a drive for longevity through the care and feeding of others. it's a healthy expression of mankind.

The scrawled "Who am I?" on the schoolyard fence may seem bizarre to some, but it's the oldest question known to civilization. **Self Identity** is the quest of every man, woman, and child. Those who struggle with it during adolescence and come up with an acceptable answer will make greater strides in life than those who fail the first test. Some of us keep questioning even after we've reached the answer—we tend to doubt its veracity for a number of reasons. Others accept an answer too quickly and never reach into their untapped potential. The answer to "Who am I?" probably changes a little every day until we pass on.

Anyone who has stood up to the crowd and became known as their own person, knows the definition of ***autonomy.*** This is a need to be independent, free of encumbrances, and not in anyone's pocket. The person with autonomy keeps the process open, despite the hue and cry for action—doesn't just stand there, does something. An autonomous individual keeps the wolves at bay because planning is needed before action, and the best plans are made with input from the people involved in the process whether at school, work, or home.

Adolescence is a risky time of life. Teenagers seem ready to try almost anything that their elders decry as foolish, thoughtless, or dangerous. They are expressing their need for ***initiative.*** Taking risks is a calculated effort when performed within limits of good sense and adventure. When properly developed, it can be seen in adults who start businesses, bring out new products and services and in general aren't put off by the lethargy and bureaucratic shuffling of others. They'll gamble a little to move the process to a better place. They'll start something and probably finish it, or get someone else to.

The last need of initiation is linked to the first need of clarity. When one is clear about the expectation, the procedures and results, it becomes a calculated risk—not a leap from a 10-story building, but a planned act of extended energy. So, too, are the other needs (and subsequently, the skills) interrelated. While each is separate and distinct as part of the human infrastructure, harmony exists only when all fit together and sing from the same sheet of music.

You've felt yourself going with a hunch, having it payoff, and then seeing the rationality of your selection in retrospect. That's your intuitive side at work, mainly. Mainly because a hunch is an inclination to close the process based on Erikson's description of generativity—leaving things better than what you found it, or creating a climate for things to get better. As such, the decision, while intuitive, does include some of your experience that says it's good to do things for more than the short term. It's a broader concept than simple decision-making.

CREATIVITY AS A DISCIPLINE

Albert Einstein, who himself was a late bloomer, recognized that creativity was the product of a complex set of traits. In short, Einstein believed it was the ability to flip back and forth between the rational and intuitive that produced creative outcomes. The facility of how one does this determines his or her creative ability.

What he's saying then is that some people tend to be more left-brained creative—engineers, accountants, doctors, lawyers and such, while others are right-brained creative—artists, musicians, writers, and so on. Those who are equally facile—left and right, rational and intuitive—are the architects, politicians and educators. These delineations, of course, are not mutually exclusive. Some politicians can't count well; some educators can't manage; some lawyers are as irrational as some writers. But the tendencies are valid.

The act of creativity, discovery of a new solution or expression for current or recurring conditions, then is a whole brain process, if Einstein was right and many agree he was.

Erikson's developmental stages led to character or trait building. For instance, the rebelliousness of adolescence is linked to what he termed Self Identity. Young people are searching for themselves, then look around themselves and see a status quo that disturbs them, so they rebel. Not having enough talent to do it effectively, they tend to make a mess of it. They make noise, become punkers, argue or pout, or do drugs.

Parents, who know about this stage, could take care to use those data for the good of the kid. The identity crisis that begins in adolescence is an opportunity for learning of both sides. (If the lesson isn't learned, it often recurs later and is known as mid-life crisis, an identity problem of a different kind.)

Learning is a high priority in adolescence even though it may not seem so to some parents. As young persons go through the period of life that brings about the greatest changes they'll ever experience, they exhibit wild swings between absolute confidence and utter despair. The energy generated during this stage of life goes unmatched compared with other stages.

Adolescents look at society and want to change the entire world—immediately. As they get in their 20s, they feel they can certainly change their culture. In their 30s, they want to change their spouse and children. Advancing to their 40s, they realize that changing themselves is a difficult and often unrewarded process. In later years, Erikson says, they reflect on what might have been and lean on a crutch resembling despair.

Not all people follow this pattern of addressing wide-sweeping, global issues and then settling for more reasonable ones before gradually coming back to self, where the greatest influence can be exerted. But many do.

In Figure 3.3 is illustrated how the sphere of influence looks and what it means in terms of change. The large area at the top of the cone is where issues such as war, peace, poverty, famine, etc. reside. These issues affect all of us to one degree or another. In the middle of the cone are the issues of career, finances, community, and so on that also impact our lives but in a way that we can reach and be involved, although not completely in control. At the bottom are the self or personal issues such as diet, defensiveness, optimism, drugs, etc., the issues over which we alone master.

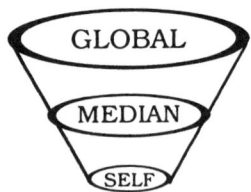

Figure 3.3. Illustrated sphere of influence.

HOW PEOPLE USE THEIR INFLUENCE

Albert O. Hirschman of Princeton wrote the book, *Shifting Involvements*, which describes how this sphere of influence cone works in real life. He studied the country's great and wealthy families, recording how they went up the cone and back down.

An immigrant, for example, comes to this country, works diligently, makes his fortune, and turns it over to the family before departing. The heirs rarely start at the bottom, but by virtue of great wealth and position begin higher up in the cone. They fail to find satisfaction working on lesser issues so gaining more power attempt to influence larger national and world problems. They continually shift their involvement searching for satisfaction that rarely comes until they retreat to their garden or study for time with nature and themselves. The Kennedys, Rockefellers, Harrimans, etc. are prime examples of these shifts.

Hirschman did not believe this has to be the case. He believed American can find satisfaction at work and at home, if they plan for it. Otherwise, he said, they'll continue the senseless quest for something that is meant to be elusive.

To develop a philosophy as suggested by sociologist Hirschman begins with knowing at least your core values, the skills necessary to achieve the level of security, status, and influence you desire, and some balance between rationality and intuition so you know when satisfaction has been reached.

ANOTHER PLACE, ANOTHER VIEW OF INFLUENCE

Ned Herrmann, who studied reality of technical professionals at General Electric for 25 years, believed the balance of left and right brain abilities is essential to the good life—satisfaction from what we do. In a nutshell, his belief is that unless a person gets in touch with feelings—the right hemisphere—he or she will be destined to only partial satisfaction, which means little at all. It's like the person who is constantly accommodating, never pushing the process to a better point. They don't appear lazy, but in fact are.

Apathy, lazy irresponsibility, or whatever label you put on it is a matter of lack of energy. Theorists put the energy source in the right hemisphere of the brain. Karl Pribram, director of Stanford University's Institute on Neurological Studies, became interested in the human infrastructure when, as a brain surgeon, he uncovered its hologramic capabilities.

Pribram's work becomes relevant to parents and teachers with adolescents because it may be the key that unlocks the direction energy is apt to take. Some call it willpower, others call it concentration or focus. For this explanation, let's call it synergy.

Synergy is a concept that originated in science when two different cells were united to form a third, better cell. Since then synergy has been observed and defined in virtually every walk of life. Teachers see it in a pupil who has the veil of understanding lifted in a course of study; a mother sees it when returning home from a short trip she finds the house in order, the kids doing homework and a stew for dinner softly gurgling on the stove; a child experiences it when crossing the street safely for the first time alone; and so on.

Everyone experiences synergy from time to time—getting more out of what you put into it or expected to get back—but few people think to plan for it. It's plannable!

Synergy is a matter of connecting loose ends or pieces. Inside the brain, Pribram saw that electrical impulses course through the corpus callosum, the bridge between the hemispheres—with an almost rhythmic regularity. This music of the mind can be symphonic, cacophonous or catatonic, depending on the mental health of the individual.

Healthy people, those with a well developed sense of themselves, use both sides of their brain interchangeably. They access the energy within themselves and develop their own kind of beat. They march to the tune of the drummer that makes the most harmony for them. Rather than plod ahead, they sometimes strut, sometimes jaunt, and usually quickstep. They also can make their movements into a waltz or a foxtrot. It's the versatility of a synergistic person that's so appealing.

ADULTS AS LEARNERS AND TEACHERS

They're in command, even in pressure and stressful situations. It's the ability to influence their own actions that deserves attention here.

George Pfaff's grandfather founded Wheelabrator Corporation in Mishawaka, Indiana more than 50 years ago. The company became the leader in its metal cleaning industry, long before ecologists talked about clean air and water with such fervor. The Pfaff family life was as wholesome as it was unspectacular.

Grandpa Pfaff brought over to this country a process to deburr and polish castings and forgings that he learned in the old country and fashioned it into a nice, comfortable little business. Things being what they were during World War II, the business expanded and developed new methods and machinery to clean slabs, billets, and other basic steel products. The difference in the Pfaff company was that it didn't use acids and chemicals like the previous technology but was a airless, blast cleaning concept—wheels within a machine hurled a b-b-sized abrasive at the steel knocking off the unwanted burrs. Thus the name Wheelabrator.

Because this methodology made a lot of dust, the company developed "dust bags" to capture particulates before they went out in the community air. The dust capturing devices grew in sophistication until this sideline eventually came into its own when air pollution became a national interest in the 1960s.

What's important about this story is that unlike some other industries at that time—steel, automotive, machine tools, etc.—didn't learn from its own markets. The Pfaff family did and sold a majority of its holdings to others until it became Wheelabrator-Frye, a substantially profitable company listed prominently on the New York Stock Exchange.

They didn't get too big for their pants, as the saying goes. The family sent young George to Notre Dame where he majored in business and marketing and brought even newer ideas to the company before it decided to cash in its chips and shift their involvements. With the solid base established by Grandpa Pfaff, and by listening to George's new ideas, the company continues as the leader in its field based on a simple philosophy—listen to customers and build to their specifications.

This simple lesson goes unheeded for a lot of adults in business, schools, government, labor and, unfortunately, at home. Parents because of their size, authority, responsibility, and position in the hierarchy tend not to be good listeners.

A common complaint voiced by some parents and reiterated by a recently interviewed father was that his first son was not at all like the second, who apparently "turned out" better. Unlike baked goods, children do turn out to be different. Each has unique characteristics, interests, and capabilities—a different set of specifications, if you will.

Malcolm Knowles of North Carolina is considered one of the foremost critics of adults as learners and his books on the subject are nonpareil. Knowles believes you can't tell adults anything—you have to make them experience it. He means, of course, that lecturing to adults is not the best way to get through to them. (It's not the best way to get information across to anyone, for that matter.) Impatient parents, who want to lump the brood into one basket and make it easier, must take the time to experience each child for what he or she is worth.

Knowles understands that Americans are a product of their schools, which have been heavily lecture-oriented. Studies as far back as the 1950s brought this to bear. (Dr. Ralph Nichols at the University of Minnesota found that we remember only 25% of a lecture immediately after and keep forgetting more each day until most of it is lost after two weeks!) Telling someone something rarely has an impact unless it's an emergency and you yell FIRE. Even then, some people will stand and stare back at you like you're crazy or something.

Lectures, of course, have a place. It affords a good listener to gain an insight into something new. Lectures also are a good preamble for a focused discussion. Lectures alone, though, have limited value. Knowles believes we should all become androgynous learners—using both hemisphere of the brain.

Giving someone a book or showing them a movie is a second favored way of disseminating knowledge. Again, the beauty is in the eye of the beholder and not everyone sees the same connotation in the written word or the projected image. In many cases, that's okay. But with a movie or a book, it's vital to allow time for the individual to process the information and then share it later in open discussion. We want people to get what they need out of an experience, but if the intention is to steer the learner to a specified conclusion, books and movies are not the best methods.

Why? Teachers don't always do a professional job of allowing time for individual, then group process. Content can create growth and stimulate thoughts and feelings but without a predictable outcome. And, that's not always bad.

Another part of the education process involves the cognitive/affective school. This had the makings of a breakthrough. The idea was to allow the learner to see something and then respond to that visual event with its affect on him or her. This works well in practice where you have a facilitator as a teacher. In those cases where you don't and that often is most of the cases, the process falls down.

WHEN ALL ELSE FAILS

What will work, however, is experiential learning. Which is to say, you have someone do something and examine the experience as soon after as possible to see what they got out of it. For instance. It's Sally's first date. She and Jimmy go to a movie, have a burger and coke after, and sit on the porch until time to come in. As a parent, you want to share in that experience as soon as you can to see if

1. Sally enjoyed herself,
2. Sally is living out the family values, and
3. Sally can express those values willingly and openly.

If you've had a good, ongoing relationship with Sally, she may want to come in, sit down, and tell you all about it. Like in *Father Knows Best.* Or, she may want to relish it and tomorrow morning may be the better time to have the chat. If you don't have a good relationship, it may be a good time to start it. Or it may already be too late.

Why it may be too late is that experiential learning is a duality of effort—it combines both thinking and feeling. If you don't have a deep-felt relationship at this stage of the developmental process with adolescent children, they know that. You probably only have an intellectual one. These single-dimension relations are all to prevalent today in this country. You can talk and be understood, but not believed.

Sally's specifications are hers alone. If you as parent and teacher have been an enabling adult, you've listened to her and can have meaningful dialogue. If you get an answer of "Out!" to the question "Where have you been?" then you've probably lost the battle and the war.

Knowles is of the belief that adults have the more difficult time learning and they have the more serious problem when it comes to bringing up their young. Adults, for some unknown psychological reason, think they have to know all the answers, be "super" moms and dads, and not show honest feelings. When just the opposite is necessary for complete family growth.

Dad may be a corporate vice president or a world beating construction worker, but he's also a man with worries, doubts, and sensitivities. He's also a man with a lot of love in him. If he withholds one set of feelings, what's to say he'll not get trapped into withholding love—another set of feelings. A lot of men in America have been socialized into hiding their feelings. The big boys don't cry syndrome. And it's too bad.

MEN AGAINST WOMEN—ONE MORE TIME

Males suffer greatly from this lack of display of their emotions. This suppression results in ulcers, heart problems, cancer, hemorrhoids, and a variety of psychosomatic ills that result in divorce, child and wife beating, career disintegration, and worse. They also inflict more long-term grief on their family—the unloved ones.

Females, although better socialized at expressing feelings, fall into some of the similar traps as the males do. Instilled with a nurturing disposition from birth through role modeling and societal expectations, today's new woman is caught in yet another double bind. If a career woman, she's also held accountable for wifely and family duties. This puts a lot of pressure on her. If not a career woman, she's often caught up in fear/guilt mode, which is also stressful and demoralizing.

A married couple attempting to work out the vagaries of their own relationship are bound to run into additional problems raising offspring. Some people work it out well. Many don't. And it's not because they don't try. They do. They simply don't have all the equipment nor the training. The bell-shaped curve on family happiness is devastated these past two generations, if you believe the statistical evidence of divorce and substance abuse as two critical criteria.

Research done a few years ago in connection with a book to be published by McGraw Hill on dual career couples discovered that while males could intellectually go along with the women's liberation movement, few could do so emotionally. The Response and Associates survey of more that 200 married couples across the country cited loss of status (power and control) as the biggest hang-up men had in creating equality in the home.

They could abide by many of the behavioral changes—helping with meals, child care, and sundry other homemaking duties normally ascribed to the wife—but struggled vainly with the relinquishing of head of household honors. Psychologists tell us this is an emotional, a feelings dilemma. Not having the experience or education of how to deal with feelings, many men retain a less than mature approach to issues of equality.

KEEP THOSE CARDS AND LETTERS COMING

Education is a lifelong process, according to Knowles and hundreds of other reputable educational sources in industry and government. On the business front, people are being replaced by machines at unprecedented rates. They need to be retrained. When word processing came on the scene in the 1970s, horrified office workers threw up their hands and declared the sky was falling down on them. Today, a company without word processing is like a cave man in the Ice Age.

The sky not only did not fall, but it increased white collar productivity for the first time since the electric typewriter.

On the personal side of it, learning or adapting yourself to changes in reality is a major challenge of the Technology Era. As systems and systems approaches become bywords in work situations, a corollary is being made with people in relationships at home. At the spiritual level, too, there is a way to bring about a more integrative approach to learning. The bible story about sowing and reaping is an example.

The sower can be seen as the teacher, the one bringing the information. The seeds that are sown are the truths. The disciples of these truths are students of life and they learn according to their ability to understand and make use of the knowledge.

Some, according to the story, do so and reap 30-fold. These are the ones who apply the literal or intellectual meaning of these data. Others reap 60-fold—they are taking the truths at a deeper, more emotional level. They have strong feelings about what they've learned.

A certain percentage of the learners, though, reap 100-fold. These are the crusaders, the one who will not only understand the message and feel strongly about, but they will march for these convictions. They are the good ground on which the seeds are sown.

The story also tells about some of the seeds falling on the roadside and being taken up by the birds. These are the emotionally insecure (flighty?) who having heard truth cannot come face to face with it and flee from dedication and duty. They have no spiritual anchorage and cannot be expected to do more until they become better grounded like the crusaders. It's going to take some risks to reach that place.

REACHING A STATE OF BALANCE

Novelist John Irving took a calculated risk 15 years ago. Rather than try and write part-time while working at another job, he put all his eggs into the writing basket and came out a winner, despite ten years of meager existence. A calculated risk. Daredevils in all walks of life weigh the prospects of one option against another and risk it. They measure their chances for success against the odds.

What generally sways the balance of these life and career choices, one way or another is the emotional satisfaction to be gained. Oh, sometimes it's money, other times it's the logical thing to do. But mainly it's ego satisfaction that controls the option to be selected. That's a good news, bad news situation.

Good news is if the odds have been shorted by a thoroughly exhaustive examination of the possible outcomes and a certain level of maturity is involved in the process. Bad news is if the selection is made with only cursory looks at it and not enough emotional discipline is at work.

For example, teenagers who yearn to compete in the Olympics often leave home for extended periods of time, live with another family near a distant training site, all with the hope of making the team. No guarantees are given, but they feel the risk is worth it. They give up friends, family, and the usual comforts of living at home to get into a 10 or 12-hour-a-day grind practicing gymnastic, skating, swimming, or track or field techniques.

These are calculated risks. They know the down side going in and what is possible should they win the gold. Still, deep down inside is a feeling that triggers their choice. Ralph Keyes, in his book, *Is There Life After High School*, described it as a status drive. Only so much status is around for teenagers and those with a chance to get their share take it whenever possible.

For dopers or drunks, status seems elusive and it appears to them that they don't seem to be getting their share. It's why their assessment of the risk—doing drugs—is worth it. They get status when they're artificially high.

Like the crusaders, the calculated risk-taker does so with full devotion. John Irving didn't quit after his first three novels failed to stir the literary world. Indianapolis 500-mile race drivers don't take the course with their hands on the brake. The opening of a Broadway show is not performed by understudies. Like other champions, the winners and crusaders reduce the risk and then give their all.

Championship football teams prepare the Sunday game plan all week to take out the bugs and doubt. The Broadway performers rehearsed their routines and lines for weeks including opening on the road to pull the product together. Race car drivers began on the dirt tracks and back roads before they pulled the throttle on the big cars. They all reach for excellence through rehearsal.

How many people do you know that rehearse? How many professionals in industry, government, schools, hospitals, stores, and shops actually take the time to go through their game plans. Some do. Not enough, but some do. They keep up to date in a variety of ways.

How many parents do you know who exercise or even have this prerogative?

MUSIC TO YOUR EARS

William Least Heat Moon wrote that a man becomes his attentions, and if that's so, then Edward Kennedy Ellington was music. The man made music his life—he paid quality attention to it from classical piano to jazz to rhythms in between—and vice versa. The Duke got high on his work.

While playing a dance gig at Indiana University in the mid 1950s, he told an interested bus boy that he liked to write a chart immediately when the idea came into his head. *"It's a balance of the moment,"* he said, sipping a cup of coffee, while jotting notes on a chart. Sam Woodyard beat his way through a drum solo and as the staccato reached its peak, Duke folded the notebook, smiled his thanks to the bus boy for the coffee and returned to the backstop, repeating to the microphone, *"Sam Woodyard ... Woodyard ... Sam."*

Many people like music in their lives. We use it as background at work, on telephone hold lines, a respite from dull and dreary moments, a reminder of Nature's harmony. It's best lesson, if we heard correctly what Duke Ellington said, is that it can be the balance of life's many moments. Whether we write it or play or just listen to it, music is a model for success in what we do.

Music is holistic. It's part rational—one, two, three, four—and part feelings—mmmm, ummm, mmmm. Equal parts of each over a time line. Whether you prefer rock and roll, waltzes by Strauss, metaphysical strings, pop ballads, West Coast jazz, or bluegrass, you keep up with the beat at two levels at least: Whether you tap you toes or move rhythmically or get up and move like mad, you're exercising one of the best means to get your head and heart together—your personal rhythm going.

It's not surprising that the major religions rely on music to keep their congregations involved and enthusiastic. People and music are inseparable. Made for each other. It's a major reason the radio, television, and live entertainment industry is one of the continuing and flourishing in this and other countries around the world.

Little words and music can reverse the most horrendous day we've had, relax the most anxious of us, and send us into a dream world of fantasy and hope. Getting into music can be uplifting, therapeutic, and just plain fun. It can be a very practical way to keep on top of things. A string is attached, of course. Drugs and music are also longtime friends.

The history of the music industry is filled with horror stories. It's performers, groupies, and executives have been most prominent in the use and abuse of substances since the first drum was beat on and the first horn blown into. Today, the rock and roll era personifies the worst of the drug scene. Its stars—Janis Joplin, Jimmi Hendrix, and others—drew notoriety by their deaths associated with overdoses. Others make headlines going in and out of treatment centers—almost as if the clearing out process was part of the business.

Not all performers and those associated with the entertainment field do drugs. They get the headlines, because their lives depend on public awareness. Maybe they get too close to the truth through their music and can't stand being too far away—a case of overindulgence. Who knows?

SUMMARY

Home is where the hat is and the values system is created for adolescents. Home is the first place of learning basics and even the more complex components of a lifelong philosophy. We know this, but few parents have a laid out plan to follow specifics over a child's various growing up phases.

Erik Erikson provided us with a blueprint.

The more we learn, the better off we are. We can't ever quit learning. Sometimes it's risky business. Calculated risks are adult choices.

Synergy is a concept, that when practiced, makes beautiful music—just like Duke Ellington.

CHAPTER 4

LIVING ON THE EDGE

Tommy Ward looked out the window. The sunlight glinted off the pane and made stripes across his bedspread. He dressed hurriedly but the stripes continued to keep his attention and he stooped to look closely at them. **"Prison,"** he thought. **"That's what it must be like in prison."** He was late for his Babe Ruth League game and he shoved his glove and shoes in the duffel bag, tossed on his cap and went banging out the door, yelling, **"See you later, Mom. Got a game."**

Shaking her head, Mrs. Ward didn't bother to answer. She knew her words would fall on a fleeing back. She promised herself to have a talk with Tommy later, when he got home at supper time. **"It would be nice, too, if his father joined in the conversation,"** she told herself. **"A boy 14 needs a father to talk man and boy talk. It's a pretty shaky time for a youngster, and a mother, well, a mother can talk about some things, but not man and boy talk."**

The ringing telephone interrupted her thoughts and she heard Tommy's father say, **"Won't make it for dinner tonight, Ellen. Got a problem here and I'll have to babysit it through. Don't worry about me—I'll get something from the cafeteria. See ya later, Hon."**

After hanging up, Walt Ward wondered if he did the right thing in taking a lateral move this late in his career. Guys his age were firmly in place in other industries. Machine tools, though, were under the gun. Foreign competition forced economy moves and he felt threatened.

Alone again, Ellen Ward wondered if she made the correct decision to stay home after Tommy was born. Her career was just taking off as a systems analyst—two promotions and three hefty pay raises in the last few years at Parker Digitronics. They were grooming her for management. Just when it looked like the world was turning right, she got pregnant. **"One of life's elegant surprises,"** *she told Walt.*

He said, **"Well, you've got options, you know. Whichever you choose, I'll support it."**

"We'll have the baby, Walt. We both want a family, a small one. And I can decide afterwards if I want to postpone my career," *she remembered saying then.*

"Some postponement. I wouldn't recognize Parker anymore. They've grown and the whole high tech world has changed so much. I'd be like little girl lost," *she told herself with a wry smile and a return to preparing dinner for two.*

Erich Fromm has written that the individual, who seeking freedom from dependency, often sacrifices one set of bonds for another. Just as the adolescent attempts to cut the ties of what is perceived as stifling authority, the inexperienced teenager draws another set of ties around—doubt and fragmented security.

In the rush toward adulthood, the awakening within the adolescent poses a double edged sword. It can be hugely exciting and grossly intimidating. Knowing that failure is not fatal, adolescents can be spontaneous, i.e., freely use their will power, their choices of integrated thought and feeling. Those who manage to learn from the excitement reach the young adult years with a spirit that contains an integration of their intellectual and emotional capabilities and potential. It's the only way of getting a natural high.

Getting high is a human ambition. We are a striving animal. We are born into it naturally. As a newborn, we are encouraged to talk, walk, and gradually take care of our own needs. We become toilet-trained, we feed ourselves, tie our own shoe laces, and who can forget the first time he/she dressed himself/herself for school. The child may have forgotten but the parents didn't. It was a natural high.

As adults we climb mountains everyday. Martin Luther King, Jr. told his audiences that he had climbed the mountain in his mind and had seen the other side. President John F. Kennedy received more than 800,000 responses to his call for the Peace Corps from America's young people. These young people saw Kennedy's mountain and wanted to get up on it and serve, asking not what the country could do for them.

Mountain tops give us a better view of the landscape. We're on top of things around us. We're nearer to God, in a sense. Having reached the top is usually a calming, serene experience being there in the solitude and magnificence of nature. The blueness of the sky, the whiteness of the clouds, the greenness of the vegetation, the black and brown ground with its hard supportive rock and soft productive silt . . . "the purple mountain majesty." The rush of the churning waters become streams for refreshing man's soul.

The mountain is high, cliffs are steep, the climb is an adventure. The descent can be safe and thoughtful. Or it can be sudden and disastrous. Those addicted to drugs know the devastation of the fall.

A song of the 60s, popularized by the Peter, Paul, and Mary, had double meaning lyrics and told a double-barreled story of the times—"Puff, the Magic Dragon" sounded to some like a fairy tale, while it was a draconian horror story for others. Ingestion of drugs was part of the "flower children" culture, a counter-culture that planted seeds for today's wasted generation.

The children of the peace-seeking 60s generation are now in the schools, the detention homes, the treatment centers, the prisons. You might say they are the bread that was cast on the waters and some came back a little soggy. Not all. Some came back nice and toasted. The sins of the fathers (and mothers) are waged on the children.

THE TREATMENT OF THE THRILL REALITY

In California, for example, youthful convicts of crimes with drug-related factors receive treatment unique to the penal system. Five of the 11 California Youth Authority (CYA) institutions provide substance abuse therapy for prisoners with alcohol and drug connections. Two are for female offenders and three are for young men. The drug therapies differ at each institution, but the program at El Paso de Robles School is worth a closer look.

Prisoners, ranging in age from 16 to 21, are housed in a cottage setting. The drug cottage is called Los Osos after the town of the same name located nearby. The cottage is similar to the college dorm—wards of the state sleep in dormitory surroundings, study in a rec room set-up, and in good weather have an expansive yard in which to exercise and lounge. At first impression, it could pass for a college campus. With one important exception—the walls are permanent and fortified.

The program in Los Osos is a court-mandated six to nine months during which the wards are under treatment for their substance abuse. The remainder of their sentence is spent in other cottages or in the state's highly acclaimed forest fire fighting program.

While the El Paso de Robles School is just that—an educational experience for young offenders—it offers a
". . . relevant and realistic program structure that allows hard core drug and alcohol addicts the opportunity to gain insight into their problems and make significant change from a life of obsession and crime to one of sobriety and responsibility." The program description reads as follows:

> Los Osos Cottage is an open dorm, six to nine month program designed to treat and aid the substance abuser in his recovery. Utilizing the theory, language and process of Reality Therapy and incorporating aspects of the 12 steps of Alcoholics Anonymous and Narcotics Anonymous, the individual is supported in his initiative to confront/change the dynamics of his substance abuse. The individuals own desire, intensive therapy, lecture/discussion, a curricula, volunteer network participation and involvement in public service work are utilized as vehicles to promote this redirection. Designed to foster

personal awareness of addiction, recognition of an establishment for a realistic life plan, the program requires the individual to accept total responsibility for his actions and ongoing commitment to recovery.

While that may seem like a mouthful of high-sounding platitudes to some, the CYA program at Los Osos Cottage is working better than one might expect. The program is good, the people running it are better.

Two groups of faculty are at Los Osos. The first is comprised of state employees. Greg Lowe, a former basketball and soccer player and coach, heads the treatment team and supervises the teaching staff. He's a nitty gritty guy with a cordial if not warm personality that is suited for managing diverse forces in an institutional setting. Greg is the right guy in the right place.

THE OTHER SIDE OF THE COIN

On the other side of the treatment coin is the consulting team. This is the group that is in the trenches . . . in close daily contact with the wards. They apply the "intensive" aspects of the therapy program. It's a no-holds barred, no stone unturned system—personal and pointed. Bill Degnan is the substance abuse coordinator. At least that his working title on the CYA business card. In reality, he's the fire that brings heat to the human malleability process. The changing of engrained behavior takes an awesome amount of human and spiritual energy.

Bill Degnan has an abundance of both. He's disquieting to be around. You never quite get relaxed around him. He's the kind of person that creates an environment for change. His enthusiasm is not contagious, it's fulfilling. Next to him the Don Knotts What Me Nervous character seems like Charlie Chan taking a nap.

After 20 minutes, you know Bill Degnan is going to make something happen. This is a personality that's needed for the tough and tricky reality. By the time these young people reach Los Osos, they've seen much of what the penal system has to offer—blase is their middle name. *"Sure, sure, I'll promise you just what you want to hear. Just get me out of here."*

The jailhouse promise and remorse are endemic to the population. Yet recitivism remains about 90% for most institutions. It's a revolving door in every state in the union. While the results are not complete at Los Osos, a betting man would like the odds on the Degnan approach.

ANOTHER TIME, ANOTHER SETTING

This program is not the first time the penal system has taken the gloves off and gotten confrontive with alcohol and drug addiction. These are the leading triggers for crime in America. The federal authorities allowed another crusader to hit the issue hard when Dr. Martin Groder set up a train-the-therapist program at its maximum security facility in Marion Illinois in 1970.

Groder used a similar mix of ingredients to formulate a new reality by recruiting convicts, serving 20 years or more and unlikely to do anything but spend the rest of their lives behind bars, to provide other penal institutions with drug and alcohol counselors. A con, who in essence had nowhere to go for quite a spell, could become productive by helping other cons rehabilitate themselves. The program was so successful—a 12% recitivism rate—the government opened a new research facility in Butner, North Carolina, under the aegis of Dr. Groder.

Like Degnan, Groder came to his vocation under strange circumstances. Groder had a four-year service liability to Uncle Sam and rather than wear a uniform, he selected the public health arena as his service. Sometimes you win, and sometimes you lose. Groder got assigned to the federal penitentiary in Marion. Oh My. He'd be behind bars for this four-year stint.

Part of the orientation to his new post as chief of health programs and chief psychiatrist was a session in San Francisco to take part in the Synanon Game for drug addicts. Because Groder had studied with Eric Berne, M.D., founder of the Transactional Analysis Seminars, he had wondered if it was possible to integrate these two powerful methodologies.

When he got to Marion, and decided to make the best of it, he formed a coalition with the support of the psychology department at Southern Illinois University and together with a handful of faculty and graduate students like Vic Green, Ted Harrison, Jim Stuart, Joe Vinovich and others designed a program based mainly on the Synanon Game and Transactional Analysis (TA). They called their enterprise the Asklepieion Therapeutic Community and Training Institute, based on the name of the physician and mythical Greek god of medicine, Asklepios.

According to legend, people who were confused or hurting came to Asklepios' temple and he spoke the truth to them while they were entranced. When they awoke from their depth experience, they knew the truth about themselves and went on their way as new men. At Marion, behind the high walls, inmates, staff and people in general can come to hear the truth about themselves and each other. They can experience themselves at a depth beyond that provided by Asklepios. Such an experience, they say, enables a man to go his way avoiding self-created walls or hiding within his self-limiting sanctuaries.

One of the major differences between Marion and Los Osos is that the hardened criminals, who are learning to be counselors, wear the same clothes, live in the same wards, have no special privileges and have undergone the same therapeutic experiences they now ask their cellmates to accept.

Like Los Osos, Asklepieion is for those who have driven themselves to the depths of despair—it's an opportunity for rebirth and, for some, a chance to learn and internalize new skills. Both are reality-based experiences that can change lives and lifestyles.

ON THE PERSONAL SIDE OF IT

For Bill Degnan, it's a second or maybe last chance. He was a civil rights activist in the 1960s. As a Catholic priest, he saw his duty and service to God clearly—defend and assist the defenseless. However, he became disillusioned with his Church and quit. Now married with a family, he's a recovering alcoholic.

He can speak with conviction about addiction. He knows what it was to be on top of the mount and how hard and bitter the fall is.

But no bitterness remains today. His lifestyle is exemplary. Although profusing energy like the crusader he is, he maintains remarkable balance. Still a tendency exists is to be the "street-fighting pastor" but in the main, he's come to grips with his own reality. He uses the principles and guides of William Glasser, M.D., the founder of Reality Therapy, and amalgamates that with his own insights and brand of no-nonsense therapy.

Instead of taking to the pulpit, he practices what he teaches. He runs for 45 minutes over the lunch period, keeping a hard, trim look about him. He fights a tendency to overweight as he fights his alcoholism—with quiet resolution and discipline. His new lifestyle suits him fine. The same goes for his staff.

One of them is no-hit fame, former baseball major leaguer Doc Ellis. The tall, fire-balling right hander pitched for seven years in the big time with the Pittsburgh Pirates, New York Yankees, and Oakland A's, before bowing to the curves of cocaine. This was also a seven-year episode that set a new course in life for him.

As a part of the Los Osos consulting team, Ellis talks to the kids in their language—he grunts, groans, and writhes his way through the abyss of addiction and brings clarity to his adolescent listeners for their struggle to get straight and clean.

Ellis tells about his fall from the mountain top. And the kids listen. So do the adults. he knows how to keep the other guy honest. Like Sal The Barber Maglie, Ellis wasn't reluctant above giving his opponent a close shave. He's been compared to Hall of Famer Bob Gibson on the mound—a Black man with a fierce desire to win. He keeps the desire to win right there on his sleeve.

Even today, he pushes the process to its most confrontive best. It's his way of putting his life back together, one piece at a time. In his baseball team-oriented way, Ellis combines his own ongoing rehabilitation with the young addicts he serves—a synergistic solution.

In this new team setting, it looks like a winning combination. They've all worked in the bottom of the pit—Groder, Degnan, and Ellis—and know how dirty it gets and how to clean up messes.

A POET IN OUR MIDST

One of the wards at Los Osos looks like he could be a second base or shortstop prospect for the majors. Blond, stocky with a flat, hard face, Rusty Bangham has the aire of a jock. It's surprising that he doesn't go much for athletics—he'd rather be a poet. Here's an example:

Life of an Addict

Living a life of fear
is the only life I know
my eyes cry painful tears
yet I try not to let it show.
I live a life of an addict
you can see it in my style,
you can see it in my eyes
and you can see it in my smile.
I'm a man who runs from reality
silently crying out,
I'm a man who is afraid to see
what life is really all about.
I ask you for your help
yet I turn and walk away,
you say I should live for tomorrow
instead I live for yesterday.
Yelling and screaming
and crawling with pain,
the withdrawal symptoms
are driving me insane.
I need that shot
to calm me down,
to lift my feet
up off the ground.

That way I don't have
to stand on this earth,
and deal with the problems
I've had since birth.
I hide in a land
of make believe,
my intentions are good
but my actions deceive.
When I look in the mirror
my reflection's not there,
and this time
it's gone for good.
I've lost the life
I never lived,
the life
that never could.

© Rusty Bangham, September, 1986
Reprinted by permission

SNAPSHOT

As Rusty works his way through the maze of rehabilitation, his parents collect their thoughts on what went wrong. Intelligent, wordly, aggressive, and successful by almost any standard this society puts on them, they are prospects to become crusaders of a different kind. Their story is a microcosm of nearly 40% of parents in America today.

Jeannie and Dick Bangham married in the early 1970s; he was the boss of a start-up trucking company serving the high tech company's in California's Silicon Valley and she was the Girl Friday. Dick learned his business from the bottom up, is proud of that. Jeannie, who grew up on a ranch in Idaho, knew how hard work and dedication can pay dividends. She also has an entrepreneurial drive to match Dick's and solves the garden variety of problems at will.

They made a good team. Everyone said so. As Viking Freight Systems made its mark and good fortune in catering to the very special needs of the computer, chip, and specialty component products business in the Western States, the Banghams bought a horse ranch in Northern California, giving Jeannie the chance to manage a business of her own in keeping with her childhood dream.

They had two children, Rusty and Darin, adding to their jam-packed activities schedule. But they loved it. These are high energy people, who thrive on activity, fun, and excitement. The boys grew towards adolescence and the pressures mounted. Rusty's energy tended to get him into trouble. He wanted attention and found inappropriate ways to get it. These diversions led to more pressures and the Banghams fell victim to their own success formula—long hours and hard work—they became a growing national statistic. No time remained for everything anymore. The string had run out. They decided to separate and live apart.

Shortly after, Rusty's cries for attention took him over the side and he became a ward of the California Youth Authority. No amount of outside help from reform school to private psychologist could provide the solace he needed for his adolescent trials and could not communicate to his parents.

THE NEXT STEPS

Today, Jeannie has a new goal. She puts her sons as number one priority. She's decided to forego her previous ambitions and do what she can to be more involved in Rusty's rehabilitation and Darin's coming of age. Just what this means remains to be seen, but she feels confident and determined about the decision.

Dick is less certain. Still chairman of the board at Viking, he's semi-retired and in search of something. He's a youthful appearing man in his late 40s, straight forward in his approach to life, and talks about starting new enterprises to keep his hand in. How and whether they will include his children is moot.

His current life is divided between boating in the Bahamas and quiet times atop a hill in comfortable Los Altos. He's a man poised for action in a serene and almost metaphysical way. Successful businessmen tend to assume this posture at critical stages in their careers. Once one major hurdle has been cleared they regroup for yet another assault. They see mountains in their minds, too. The valley of time in between is contemplative, nature-oriented, and filled with silent energy.

PARENTS LOOK BACK AND WONDER—WHAT IF . . .

Parents have a habit of looking back and seeing things clearly from their own perspective. They review the upbringing of their children in a kind of motion picture screening. Each reel is edited according to current status, not with the turmoil and tensions of the past moment.

Fromm noted that the spontaneity of the artist is within us all, but the more rational people—those who do not immediately respond to their feelings—run a different course. They become successful in their own right. Some become the captains of industry, the political statesmen or the revolutionary of their times. Some are more limited but equally content within a given playing field. They accept the boundary and sphere of influence. The unsuccessful at adaptation become criminals.

Groder, Degnan, and other crusaders have made mistakes during the early phases of their lives. Not abject failures, of course, but they mistook the emotional aspect and put the energy in the wrong place or gear. It clanked and made a strange, unproductive noise. Somehow they listened and were able to restart their engines, driving this time with a new understanding of where they were headed.

THE PATH TO POWER IS STREWN WITH BODIES

The story in the Bible tells of Christ falling on the way to the hill on Calvary. Burdened as He was with a cross of man's sins, He got up and continued the slow march. Bill Degnan, for one, didn't trade in his old one for a new one when he left the

Church. He merely took another path up the hill. So did Doc Ellis. So may Rusty Bangham and many who have fallen down and scuffed their knees and egos.

The new crusaders are teaching a process—an inclusive, possibly more exacting path up the hill. It starts with the fall and teaches the injured how to get up, regain a balance, and walk on. They work with the fallen—the addicted of our society. Just like Christ did. He seldom went to the affluent to tell His stories, hoping to provoke change in behavior.

Crusaders seldom find the going easy. Like the artist, the crusader is vulnerable. The spontaneity involved in crusading goes against the grain. People just don't want to listen to the truth. They'd rather take a steroid instead of spending an extra hour pumping iron. They'd rather accept the doctor's prescription for yet another jar of addictive codeine than search for a cure to migraine. They want a cookie cutter—answers in a step-by-step procedure so they don't have to think or invest of themselves. So it's an uphill all the way. It's easy to forget that you want to drain the swamp when you're surrounded by alligators.

VIVA LE DIFFERENCE

The process at Asklepioein differs from Los Osos and is different from Tough Love and a myriad of other attempts at treating the addicted and those around them. While each its own tack, they all sail on the same sea. Experience has brought the process closer to port than before. They all realize that the spirit must be renewed along with the corporal self.

God knows none of the approaches is perfect. Each has built-in distractions, not to mention the distractions and other baggage people bring to the process. What these approaches have in common, though, is exciting. Unlike previous treatment therapies, they begin with the knowledge that people are in a state of powerlessness. Each of these integrative therapies start with the given. Like the good pro quarterback, they take what the defense gives them.

Today's crusaders have learned the valuable lesson that you can't correct the past nor prepare for the future overnight. Nor can you do it with wishful thinking and faulty recollections. **Addicts are out of control and require discipline to develop a new lifestyle,** including a philosophical outlook. The new therapies are designed with this in mind and the therapists are making that point clear before moving on with more clarity towards the top of the hill—towards the Supreme Power.

THE ALPHA STAGES—AWARENESS AND OPTIONS

The will to change is within us. While the television commercials shout the joys of good health through proper diet and exercise, little is proposed about carrying the commitment down to the core values. People in this age of instant gratification want "it" done to them. They want the miracle of life to continue through pills and serums and dictums.

The good news is that some of the more than 40 million health-seeking Americans—ones who daily or near so—take it in their own hands to jog, hike, bike, row, stroke this ball or that in an effort to rid themselves of debilitating stress.

The physicality of today's culture is impressive. Once considered a fashionable fad—Gucci running togs notwithstanding—the weight of the evidence (excuse the pun) is that America has adopted a cultural lifestyle that does not any longer condone hard liquor, gross obesity, and, somewhat surprisingly, flagrant promiscuity. It's in to be healthy, looking good, and more careful of your sexual activities than in the past.

Despite the fact that many people are smoking today, the Surgeon General's message is getting through—more have quit smoking than ever before. The paradox is linked to stress. The complexities of 21st century living are a tall mountain.

Because health is more than a physical phenomenon, the source of stress relief and management includes attention to mental and emotional fitness as well. The research gains in these subtle and psychological areas are not currently as great or as evident as the physical status, but progress is being made. More is in the offing. We now can certify that at least 80% of all illness and injury has a stress or stress-related facet.

By looking at what it costs American corporations for health care benefits—nearly $200 billion in 1986 and rising—you get an idea of what's going to be the focus of cost containment during the next few years. Wellness and employee assistance programs are abundant throughout Corporate America and will likely continue to grow as the evidence is counted. Healthy workers are productive ones. And people tend to take home what's going on at work, and vice versa.

Just a few years ago, critics laughed at the Japanese practice of having workers exercise and sing songs prior to the start of the work day. The Orientals have long been advocates of harmony and balance amongst the personal aspects of a clear-thinking mind, a disciplined range of emotions and a body attuned to its own well being. They've known for centuries that it's better to take the ounce of folksy prevention, rather than gulp a pound of uncertain cure.

Even today's traditional medical approaches are yielding to the holistic inroads of Eastern Philosophies. The prevailing thought amongst medical practitioners in America today has shifted from the one-sided scientific school to a more malleable one of treating the whole person—mind and emotions included. So much of illness can be linked to psychosomatic origins that most doctors recommend therapies linked to total involvement—carrying the "take two of these and rest" direction to a new level.

The merging of these two schools will benefit the society and heed the words of Thomas Alva Edison, who predicted that the work of doctors would be more of teaching people to care for themselves, rather than be passive subjects for treatment. He said: "The doctor of the future will give no medicine but will interest the patient in the care of the human frame, in diet, and in the cause and prevention of disease."

While it's too bad that the ill and the injured have forced the adaptation in medical habits, let's be thankful for the change. The injured can be the crucial catalyst for their own recovery. At least that's what Victoria Aldrich believes.

ANOTHER CRUSADER IN DISGUISE

Victoria runs a vocational rehabilitation service in Davis, California. She is a fully credentialed counselor/therapist with a master's degree and certification from the two leading institutes serving this specialized field of voc rehab. Her experiences with returning injured people back to work led her to believe that people will do what's possible to be productive and healthy, if you give them the chance. It's what makes her a success in a field frought with malingering.

As soon after an accident, that has in one way or another crippled a worker, Victoria goes to see the employee. She schedules a two-hour face-to-face interview and begins an intimate dialogue that leads the injured person to a decision point—will I get well or indulge myself with pity. Victoria's style, if you want to call it that, is professional. She's a disciplined person. Her emotions are under control. She's informed and articulate to inform the injured worker. Vicki lays it on the line and, at the same time, is open to the particular needs of the disabled.

What she listens for are the non-verbal messages. These are the hidden agenda items that often escape detection, if you're not paying attention. They are emotional signals that can best be detected on the intuitive radar of the listener. Like a dancer expressing deep-felt feelings, people give off solid information about themselves through a variety of nuances. It's almost analogous to the jailhouse promise; the often bed-ridden employee may go along intellectually with the rehabilitation program, but underneath may be all aglow with the opportunity to "get even" with the company, the supervisor, the system. Some don't get mad, they calmly and cooly get even.

One observation that Vicki makes, though, makes sense. "When someone is hurting, really in pain, they learn faster than usual. Oh, I don't mean they listen to me, their doctor, or some other authority figure quicker. I mean they dig deep down into themselves and question their very being. The answers they come up with tend to stick. If my input is in line with their values, we'll have a good recovery. And that's what happens most of the time."

The worst the injury, the more thoughtful the inquiry. *"I know people who have escaped death by inches will be the most likely to make significant changes in their lives. It's as if the close brush with death brings them nearer to their soul,"* she explains in her reserved enthusiasm.

On a more practical side of it, Vicki can tell you in 15 minutes what her chances are of convincing the worker to motivate him or herself into getting better and returning to some form of dignified and productive work. One of the big stumbling blocks she encounters is drug abusers. The injured worker may be on drugs prior to the injury, or, as is the case in an alarming number of situations, the person became addicted to drugs used in treatment.

Because of her talent, Vicki can count on a 90% to 95% success ratio with patients who don't get hooked or who aren't on drugs in the first place. With drug involvement, not even her wholesome, attentive, and nurturing skills can bring the figure to better than 50/50. That costs the company, to be sure, but it hurts the person more so. They become victims of the "disability" syndrome.

People who have a perception of not being all right, will act accordingly. In Vicki's line of work, it's possible to head it off at the pass by getting to the person as soon after the injury as possible. It's not so easy in drug or alcohol rehabilitation. Years of bad habits have been working in most of these cases. Miracle cures are not common in this field.

PULLING BACK THE COVERS ON INSIDIOUS RELATIONSHIPS

Bill Degnan calls it "chemical thinking." Where you or I would see the world in one way, the abuser sees it much differently. Abusers see it through an altered state of consciousness. They are totally focused and consumed with one passion—chemicals. They concede nothing to food, air, and even sex. The top priority is how, when, and where will they get their need met. They'll live on the edge to get satisfied.

If they are out of money, they will do whatever has to be done to get their chemicals. No value or moral judgment is involved at this moment. If they are out of contact with their regular dealer, their whole energy is trained on getting another junkie. They will walk away from family, friends, and other comforting resources to fly in the face of any danger. It's a compulsion you have to see to believe. In the words of Carlos Casteneda, they are totally into "a separate reality." It's the bottom side of the synergistic coin. They have integrated mental, emotional, and physical aspects to imbalance.

The way out of this maelstrom is by invoking a higher level of energy—the spiritual. By tapping deeper into one's reservoir, it's possible to correct the imbalances that substance abuse brings about. Skills, that once were in sync, can be brought to bear on self-realization. Through understanding one's connection to Higher Order, a revitalization can occur, which creates a clearer picture of the world and one's role in it.

The starting place is through meditation. In the contemplative posture, we can visualize how we are spending our time. Do we live in the past? The future? Or are we fortunate enough to spend most of our moments in the here and now, listening, learning, and doing spontaneously? If we look back and forward without purpose—no spiritual attachment—we tend to the sin of omission.

Those who act without reference points tend to sins of commission. These people create an imbalance, which is an insult to the balanced system. These rash acts are an indulgence like the ones perpetrated by dopers and drunks. They do so in the hope of gaining a fast-forward life. What happens instead is that continual frustration leads to sins against self.

To get out of this addictive rut the abusers need to stretch their belief system. The stretch covers primary needs to spiritual ones. This means that physical, intellectual, and emotional growth will be nurtured by the individual's universal spirit. When your car is out of gas, you go to a gas station to replenish the supply. Some people pray for replenishment, when they're on empty. Others demand it through childish squeaks and clamors—gimme, gimme. We all know those who expect the best to happen without lifting a finger; we all know people who expect the worst, no matter what.

THE ALPHA PROCESS—A STARTING PLACE

Growth, progress just doesn't happen that way. Recovery begins when the addict admits failure and begins anew. Through a calm meditative examination of consciousness—not conscience, that comes later—the vital statistics are revealed. It's not the same as going to confession and getting it off your chest; telling what you did wrong. It's accumulating the information about the current state of your well being and using these data to figure out a remedial schematic. It's more an assessment of your personal tool and survival kit. You jiggle through the people skills and technical competences, brush off the communications and teamwork abilities, and evaluate their combined impact on your bottom line.

Awareness is being alert to what's going on around you and with you. When you say something, how does the other guy react? When you say that same thing, how were you thinking and feeling? As simple as that sounds, many people simply are not aware. They have built up a series of predictable reactions to life that becomes ritualistic in nature. Some ritual is okay, but not on an exclusive basis.

Getting in touch with your own behavior after years of not paying attention is an arduous but not impossible task. Most professionals accept it as a way of life. Athletes watch movies and videos of themselves. Actors review the daily rushes. Good managers relish the feedback from subordinates and superiors alike. Prosperous companies follow Tom Peters advice and listen to their customers—even to the point of redesigning and developing new products and services.

These same professionals are not as likely as anyone else, however, do so the same thoughtful and insightful process with their personal behavior. In the old days, they called it being self-centered, ego-centered. While the tag may be inappropriate, the concept isn't. Without a centered, grounded, or awareness of self energies, the individual is apt to be as scattered as shot from a 30-ought-6. Paying attention under the stress of the moment is what's needed.

Gathering data about your own actions and intentions in one way to develop a systemic pattern. [What? You said that rituals (patterns) were not the best way to live.] A system is not a ritual. A ritual is a definite, unchanging set of ways. A system is a flexible, responsive-to-the-environment set of ways. A systemic pattern, then, is interactive—a chance to hit the target by adapting to the idea of Kentucky windage—putting it's human instinct to work to catch the way the wind is blowing.

When one becomes aware, options become apparent. Under ritualistic behavior—going to lunch with the same crowd everyday, driving to work the same route, coming up with the same solutions to old and recurring problems—there's little chance for creative applications. The door to newness is closed.

When options are uncovered, choice comes to life. With choice comes it's twin, risk. One choice is riskier than another. Some care and thought must be given to analyzing the choices and attendant risks. If the assessment taken during the awareness phase was exhaustive, the choices will proliferate. Too many choices can stifle the process and bring about "analysis paralysis."

This phenomenon can be seen in most institutions where they call a meeting to check the schedule of upcoming meetings. People can't be contacted during the workday because they are in meetings. Productive work comes to a screeching halt, while minds are numbed with rehash and massage.

To overcome this malaise, catalysts are needed to prompt the process. Options, after examination and inquiry, are set up in priority fashion. A variety of formulas are available to establish criteria for prioritizing: you'll be introduced to one in a later chapter. That's not the most important part of it anyway—pruning the list is. The prioritizing process should include a way to reduce the list to the most viable two or three choices.

That's a manageable number and one that allows for higher concentration of energies. Management is what comes next in the process, after you've made the decision. But let's look more closely at decision-making. It can petrify you, and often does just that, or can be the forum for getting the best out of all concerned.

DECISIONS, DECISIONS, DECISIONS

Promises are a decision made, yet to be fulfilled. Our lives are filled with them . . . people have a promising career ahead and fail to live up to that potential . . . a parent hints at a special trip with the kids that never comes off . . . the adolescent longs for the future when he or she will be among the rich and famous.

Without the promise, though, some decisions are put off and never gotten around to. The driving force of many decisions, then, is the extraction of a promise—a commitment to perform. This goes back to a moral and ethical aspect of human nature. It's a historical precedence that "a man's word is his bond" and this human inclination precedes our national legal system.

The Japanese, for one, do most of their business with a bow and handshake. They have only a small percentage of their professions allocated to lawyers—a practice many Americans agree would be worthwhile following.

To the Japanese, breaking your word is tantamount to "losing face," an insult to heritage and ancestry, often causing serious repercussions, some self-inflicted. In our culture, it started out that way, maybe not as self-denigrating, but certainly as morally and spiritually staggering.

Our forebears were committed to each other. Neighbors helped neighbors in a new world where the climate and adversities of nature proved calamitous. The pioneering spirit was akin to the spiritual energy that crossed the Atlantic Ocean. A natural affinity was with the Lord and only a few disregarded the obvious.

When gold was found in California in 1848 and in subsequent years "claim jumping" seemed to become a divergent practice from the norm. Instead of respecting one man's bond to a discovery site, the easy way was to steal it. Without being an apologist for the 49-ers, perhaps it was greed and a despair for the adverse nature of this country that some men put economics before self respect. Whatever the reason, this nation slowly moved from a handshaking, neighborly culture to a suspicious, contractual one.

With the move, a national heritage was moved aside, or at least further from the mainstream. Some trust was lost in the process and we moved away from Judeo-Christian principles and more towards a common law. With it came the hordes of piggling law suits that chokes our judicial system and worse, a nation indebted to economic bottom lines.

This made us into a short-term thinking nation. We make decisions based on quarterly or annual reports. As parents, we look at the latest report card, not the trends associated with child rearing. Our reactive nature, a product of short-range thinking, keeps us from developing a conceptual framework and skills needed to be far-sighted and patient.

Can we stem this slippage? Can we regain what was once a birthright in this nation? Is there the personal force to do so?

Yes. Yes. Yes.

The nation has shown a patriotic spirit in the recent past and a resurgence of spirituality. The coupling of these energies is producing a synergistic effect that, properly focused and directed, will enable thoughtful and productive people to do what's in their hearts. The national leaders are sensing it, just as Kennedy and Reagan did.

Given any definable set of circumstances, Americans are talented enough to manage even the worst of scenarios. Given a national and personal imperative, we rise to the occasion. Whether a high-paid executive for a technology firm or a homemaker with a diverse set of activities, Americans respond once the facts are known. We are good problem solvers. Our long suit is creative solutions.

That's what faces us today. The substance abuse situation is well known. While the national agenda seems temporarily overly concerned with the supply side of the issue, the pendulum is swinging toward equilibrium. That means, a balanced approach to give equal concern to the demand side—the user and abuser.

The $100-billion-plus economics of this national tragedy will not allow for an easy answer. People, who like the claim jumpers, have greed on their side will not be deterred from gross profits at the expense of human lives. They'll connive and steal and cheat like they always have, using the latest and the oldest means at their disposal—smuggling technology and low life distributors.

From now on, it's a religious war. You're either going to be on one side or the other. There are no other choices. It's a participative game from here on out. No bystanding. No popcorn sellers. No ticket takers. You're on the drug side or the side of self-respect and self-realization.

SUMMARY

Life can be a thrilling experience, sometimes with threat to life and limb. It's certainly not risk-free, but it's best experienced with all faculties in motion.

Taking care of the hurt and injured is part of the process. Taking care to reduce the number at risk is also part of it. The practitioners are giving us valuable information about what can be done to prevent a worsening of the substance epidemic.

Some parents are coming to grip with their realities. It's not easy to be a successful parent. But it's not too late to change course in the predominant number of cases.

The time is ripe for a return to pioneering practices that our forebears delineated in their battle against overwhelming odds—the forces of a wild and caustic nature.

As a nation, we're currently putting most of our eggs in the supply side of the substance abuse issue. The issue requires the equilibrium of supply and demand. The youth of America, their teachers and parents—together—are aware of the problem.

Three questions are on the table, requiring three decisive answers. These answers rest on the promises of the reader.

PART II
BECKONING...
GROWTH OPTIONS

CHAPTER 5

THE KINDRED SPIRIT

As day was turning to the dark of evening Tommy Ward knew he would catch heck if he was late again. He knew that studying with Petey and Debbi was the most enjoyable time he could possibly have with school work. Whether at his or her house, the homework took on real life meaning—it wasn't just history or geography. It was real people and places. The three of them made it alive.

They'd joke and laugh a lot, but seemed to learn as much if not more than the other kids. Teachers knew about this trio. They encouraged their common sharing of ideas, questions and study. Even when they'd start to break up the class with one of their extemporaneous skits.

Tommy wondered, for a second why getting that spirit into his own house was so difficult. His mom and dad seemed to be a damper on the study times, so the kids just alternated between Petey's and Debbi's houses. After all more room and privacy lent themselves to the trio's spontaneous self-expression.

Tommy hoped his parents wouldn't be too angry with his being late.

The philosophers from the time of Plato and Aristotle have known that knowledge is power. Most agree that the seat of power—where it's possible to accumulate tremendous energy—is the family. The family is where the personality is formed and attitudes for life take shape.

At home is where people learn those values and skills for success, joy, and happiness. Too often, it's also where distrust, frustration, and bad habits take root. If a man's home is his castle, the knight's armor mail may be rusting faster than it can be kept in clean, working order.

The statistics are alarming. More than 200,000 readers of *Better Homes and Gardens* magazine responded to a poll on the state of the family, saying, "We're in trouble." As for causes of the trouble no consensus was present—the multiplicity of it suggested no simple solution—and better than 80% were discouraged by the disintegration of the nuclear family. The poll was taken in 1983 and more recent surveys by reputable opinion pollsters indicate little has changed to correct the perception.

Divorce heads the list of most observers as the trigger for the splitting of family harmony and single parent households are growing at non-stop rates. In 1970, two-parent households accounted for 87% of family structure, while single-parent situations were at 12.9%. Ten years later, the figures were 78% to 22%. Today, the numbers are closer to 70% and 30%.

The trend, according to Senator Daniel Moynihan of New York, will continue until in the year 2000 when America will have half of its households in each category. If the philosophers are correct and most of the power comes from the integrated family, then America is cutting severely into its hope for a solid and strong future. The power may not be severed in half, but the damage is irreparable.

This is not to denigrate the single-parent household. Many, if not most of them, manage to surpass the standards of their previous nuclear standing. It's more than the lesser of two evils. A household with a drunk or a spouse as a child abusing parent is not the healthiest of places to raise a family, and so often the separation or divorce is called for. The resulting single-head of household, however, is a debilitating and a national disaster, despite the often herculian efforts advanced by the smaller family unit.

The result of divorce deprives all members of its intended power.

In America, single-head of households means mothers at the helm. Here, the trend is unmistakable. In 1970, 33% of them were headed by Black mothers and 8.9% by White mothers. In 1980, it was 48.9% Black and 15.1% White, indicating that White women were catching up in the statistics. The most recent figures are 60% of Black mothers and 20% of White mothers. Male head of households, while significantly smaller, are also growing exponentially—2.6% Black and 1.7% White in 1970 and 3.9% and 3.1% today.

Unmarried head of households, too, is on the rise, according to U.S. Census Bureau information. In 1970, the numbers were 0.3% were White and 5.4% were Black. Today, the figures are 3.4% are White and 33% are Black.

Then the relatively new phenomenon is dual career couples. This is a situation where both spouses work at a job. Some, in the case of the female, because they have to support the family and others because they want to, furthering their own self worth and career ambitions. These arrangements comprise nearly 35% of nuclear family situations and are also on the rise dramatically since 1970.

Dual career couples are another wedge driven into the sanctity of family harmony. While much has been written and said about "quality time"—better focus and attention to each other—the record is totally inconclusive as to its positive results. The record is clear on the shortcomings associated with dual careers.

For instance, even though the wife's employment brings economic assistance to the family, the time available for her as a parent is drastically diminished. The male in dual career families has not, statistically, changed enough to adopt the so-called "feminine" chores—they still struggle to maintain "head of household" responsibilities rather than shift to equality of duties.

The analysis is grim.

As a nation, we take sides on issues that emanate from this conflictful and changing family situation. For instance, one-half of us get on the pro-abortion side and one-half on the pro-life side of the argument. One-half of us see value in the Equal Rights Act and one-half don't. These and other stalemates cut heavily into our national psyche. Congress—pressured by a two-year produce or get out syndrome—spends its time and our money on legislation to attend to these issues without getting at the root causes.

Then too industries are built around the problems. Divorce lawyers abound, lobbying groups are formed, counseling centers grow, health facilities proliferate, and countless non-productive time and effort are spent reacting and coping with problems without initiating curbs or a cure.

Worst of all, this folderol is what's behind the demand for drugs and alcohol in our adolescents. They think it's all a little bit insane, and they want to have some fun—not being led around by a reactionary adult population that gets emotionally involved, flailing away at giant windmills.

WHAT'S REALLY GOOD FOR EACH FAMILY MEMBER?

Two questions are on the table in this country today. Is hope possible for the nuclear family in the near future? Can single-parent households develop into healthy, productive families? Fortunately, the answer to both is in the affirmative, but it isn't going to be easy. The patient, though, may be ready for the cure.

A little known publication in Canada, *Maclean's* magazine took a poll a year ago and asked its readers if the end of the family as we know it is in the offing. Of the respondents, 46% disagreed, while 15% strongly disagreed, or 71% felt the family could recover its former status as the bulwark of society. Less than a third agreed with the tenet and only 8% had strong convictions that the family unit was dead in the water.

Another promising signal comes from the corporation. They are now getting involved in the personal side of employees' lives and finding out that it's good, sound economic cost-effectiveness to do so. The company, government agency or institution once felt that what goes on off-duty was none of their business. Rising employee benefits costs, worldwide competition and a broader understanding of human nature has removed that look-the-other-way philosophy from the boardroom. The business of business is still business, but it extends to personal lifestyle as much as it impacts on health and performance on the job.

Nearly 90% of managers and officials of one corporation with plants and offices all over the world had one common problem that loomed over all else and that was a concern for parent/child relationships. A general manager of a $6 million operating unit couldn't talk to his 16-year-old son without losing control of his emotions and thereby ending any hope of creatively resolving a life-threatening conflict. A yuppie sales supervisor told his 14-year-old daughter he'd rearrange her teeth in the heat of the moment—the same teeth that he'd spent $3000 for the orthodontist to fix.

To look at these parents, who perform miracles at work with 50, 60, or sometimes 100 diverse and unruly people, you'd think they could control a group of three, four or six people at home. The truth is they could, if they used the same energy over the same skills that have done them so well in the work place. The trouble is they get hooked by the emotions of the family.

The trouble is they forget what they've learned at work. The trouble is they don't plan and strategize the same way in both places. While they may lose control once in a while at work, they usually do at home. But, the employer is finally coming to realize that and is attempting to do something about it.

The last sign that help for the family is on the way is that more young people are making the decision, on their own, to beat the odds. On their own means, through a variety of trial and error experiences coupled with serious educational efforts—outside the normal school system—they are opting for a more useful, creative, and worthwhile way of life. In part it's spiritual, part intellectual, part physical and part emotions—they are discovering how to have fun without drugs and booze.

THE CONNECTING OF THESE LOOSE ENDS IS SYNERGY

Russ Latham is one example. And so is his family. The family is in a dual career situation—mom is an accountant and dad runs a radiator business in Contra Costa County, California. Sociologically, they're middle to upper middle class people: hard working, strong basic values. They have a dual reward/punishment system, too. Mom gives out the bouquets and Dad metes out the discipline—a kind of typical American family.

It figured that Russ would want to follow his mother's lead and get into the accounting field. He felt closer to her than to his father because she seemed to be ready to listen when he wanted to talk. But that's getting ahead of the story. Russ Latham took off on a ten-year roller coaster ride that ended with his becoming a dope addict.

A YOUNG SHOOT GROWS INTO A WILLOW PLANT

Russ was sixteen when he noticed that he was different from other kids in school. He felt ill-at-ease in a variety of situations—awkward with girls, stumbling with teachers and put off with the guys. A good baseball player—he turned the double play with the best of his peers—he soon saw that his short stature would not serve him well in a league that was dominated by bigger, stronger and more confident boys his own age. It was the confidence issue that gnawed at him.

So he started drinking. A couple of beers before a party put him into a better frame of mind and he could at least joke and jostle with other kids. When the beers wore off, though, he found himself back in that "I'm Not Okay" state of mind. At this stage he met, Mr. R., his first role model. Mr. R. hung around Russ' school and made friends with a lot of the kids. He was a flashy dresser, had a fancy car, an easy way with the ladies and he liked Russ. Mr. R., of course, was a dope dealer.

Russ started with marijuana and soon graduated to the more sophisticated street drugs like crank, speed, and so on. His feelings of inadequacy vanished with drugs. At least, he didn't notice how awkward or stumbling he was anymore. His parents, however, did. This led to arguments and shouting matches and eventually to a family counselor. Russ would alternate going alone and with his mother.

The visits would go something like this:

"How you doing in school, Russ?"

No answer, but the defiant look of teenage would scream back and say, You gotta be kidding? What in the hell does that matter? Are you out of your goddam mind? Let me out of this place!

After six months of no-contact with the psychologist, Russ and mom went their different ways. Anyway, Russ and Mr. R. were moving up in the world and guns came into vogue. The fifth burglary resulted in arrest and a sentence to 60 days in the county prison. It wasn't too difficult to get loaded in prison, once you got to learn the ropes, and Russ began to practice what Bill Degnan earlier described as "Chemical thinking." A listen into Russ' mind at those moments and it sounded like this:

"Why does all this happen. So silly, Mom with her drinking. Dad with his. Paul with his. Me with mine. Don't they know what I want. Where does all this shit fit. Can't they see what I need and why. I can't get it. When will they get off my case and start to listen to what I'm saying or not saying and want to say and forget to say and say again. Why can't I just get loaded and leave it be at that. Time passes so slowly in this damn dirty joint. No one cares or gives a shit and I don't give a crap either for anyone here or there or anywhere. When will I get out and get clean and get straight and ain't that a bunch of shit. I want to be free and fly and be off in my world on my time and my rules and my soul is mine and no man ain't gonna get any piece large or small if I have to blow them away and someday I will so help me God. If I could only get out and get loaded, things would be fine and no one

would be hurt and the sun would shine and be just fine and I'm a poet don't you know it. Where the hell am I and why can't I just be quiet."

Russ wasn't always racing to his own oblivion. Before drinking and doing drugs, he was pretty normal, a little more frenetic than some kids, but not too many. He was impatient about growing up, sure. On drugs, though, he was bright enough to do something about it. Something was missing, but then he met Cheryl.

Cheryl liked Russ. He was thoughtful, considerate and wasn't grabby like a lot of guys were when they discovered she was divorced. She didn't mind that Russ seemed frenetic—she wrote it off as youthful energy. She liked how he looked and acted and told him so. They started dating and Russ knew she was special. Cheryl had a two-year-old child and Russ enjoyed the instant status as lover/husband/father. His brother had quit drugs when he got married and Russ figured he would do the same.

She warned him that she didn't go for dopers and Russ honestly thought about quitting. But he couldn't. Even for Cheryl and the baby.

At first he tried to hide the fact from her, but that's like trying to hide a battleship in your backyard. He'd deny it and they'd argue and finally she issued the ultimatum. *"I won't let you put the baby in this situation, Russ. If you can't shake the habit, I'm gone and that's that,"* Cheryl told him.

He didn't believe she'd leave and the jolt of finding her gone shook him deeply. It was a shock wave that reached deep into his drug-crazed brain. For a short while, he had a family—one that suited his fondest wishes—and just like that they vanished and along with it the joy and comfort that he longed for. So he went back home and tried to reconstruct his life. That worked for about two weeks and then he pushed them to the wall.

His mother and father decided he wouldn't change as long as he kept up the associations with scum bag pushers. A change of scenery seemed to be a logical move. So they arranged for Russ to visit his aunt who lived in Oregon. He went, stole from her, rolled his car, stole another and got arrested in Oregon and sentenced again. This time he had to take a drunk rehabilitation program as part of the sentence. And then, a light went off in his befuddled and drug-agonized brain.

"What are you doing here? Why are you doing this to yourself?"

Something happened at the drunk program that persisted and Russ got off booze. That helped, but it didn't connect, unfortunately, on the drug addiction. They didn't reach that part of him. One night after he got out he raced back to Antioch, got loaded with Mr. R. and drove back to Oregon with a fresh supply.

After nearly four years of stealing, mainly from his parents and relatives, Russ came up against it. His bent for accounting took him to his father's office, where he scooped up the payroll checks and went on another spree. When his father confronted him later, the scene was quiet but heavily charged with emotions.

"Russ, I've put up with all of your stuff for a long time. I know I may not have said what's on my mind when I should have said it, but I'm telling you now. I don't want to see you again. As far as I'm concerned, you don't exist," and his father turned and walked away. As he did, he brushed tears away without regard for how it looked. Al Latham felt desolate.

This rejection finally made an impact on Russ. Shortly after that confrontation, Russ enrolled in a drug rehabilitation program at Discovery House. He's learned something there that sticks with him—it seems he's survived this ordeal of growing up to make something positive out of his life.

He's been sober—off booze—for nearly four years now. He talks to teens and their parents as part of a program for first-time alcohol and drug abuse offenders in a program run by the Concord Police and the Contra Costa School district. He's very convincing in his new role as spokesperson for the drug-free community. No more awkward or stumbling pauses. He's open, honest, and lucky to be alive. He knows it and shares that with his new audience.

He's set up a book of restitution accounts to pay back the $9100 that he ripped off, mainly to his parents. His mother has quit drinking and serves on the Contra Costa County Drug Commission. His father can now put his arms around Russ and hug him. They recently gave him the code to the $3000 burglar alarm system they had installed to keep him away from their valuables.

Russ recently graduated from a two-year course in computers at Heald College and got himself a job, handling payroll for a local industrial designer. What goes around, comes around, or so they say.

Is he a crusader? He's sure on the right track today. Coincidentally, Russ is in a Nine Year—finishing up on old business. Next year is his One Year—he'll be starting on several new projects in his life, including more intensive work with would-be addicts. He thinks that prevention is the best route to follow. He also fits into a growth pattern that Erik Erikson described in his research. The developmental psychologist may have hit on a prevention principle serendipitously.

WHAT DOES ERIK ERIKSON SAY ABOUT PREVENTION?

Three of Erikson's major research works, once connected, give some food for thought about adolescent needs and growth. First, he identified the stages we all go through from birth to adulthood. Second, he worked with Navajo Indians who resisted becoming part of the White Man's culture, and third, he researched the effects of severe stress on American soldiers in combat.

Alone, each of these studies provided his colleagues with an abundance of help in working with parents and children to develop life skills; enabled greater facilitation of cross cultural adaptation, and assisted in developing workable methods for coping and managing stress. Together, the research projects provide a synergistic solution to the addiction dilemma.

Look at Russ Latham's situation in terms of Erikson's integrated research. To begin with, Russ began his drug odyssey in early adolescence by rebelling against parental authority. This is a common reaction by teens, according to Erikson, who are searching for their own identity. Erikson called it the "identity crisis" and followers have studied its implications for years.

For a variety of reasons, teenagers throughout the ages have looked at the world of their parents and rejected it out of hand as their option for what the world could be. They assume a "cultural defiance" and see the world as not sane, not ideal, and not worth following.

Today, they look at the nuclear arsenals, world poverty, the starving and homeless, and the lack of agreement on how to make the world better and, either consciously or sub-consciously, reject the notion that their life has to follow this pattern of "going along" with current policies. They become motivated to rebel, i.e., an adolescent attempt at changing the situation. Because they lack the adult skills to be effective, they become frustrated and cause their parents unsettled moments—to put it mildly.

Like the Navajo Indian, this adolescent rebellion against their culture causes them to reject the status quo and to be part of it during their self identity stage.

In Russ' case, he rebelled until he met Cheryl and then he wanted a chance to prove to himself and others that he could do a better job in raising a family to ideals that he felt within himself. Unfortunately, by this time he was addicted and couldn't do what his value system was telling him. The shock of her leaving did leave its mark though. If he couldn't have Cheryl and what she offered, he could return to his mother, the ultimate female in his world.

Mother brought the comfort and solace that jibed with his values. After all, he learned them at her knee. It was in early childhood that Russ became familiar with competence, determination, teamwork, communications, and economics—the core values he cherishes today. The family practiced them and he learned them.

The rejection by his father in the office following the check-stealing episode sent a mind-stilling shock through Russ. He reacted by asking for drug treatment. The rejection was necessary to stimulate his deep-seated values. It was a shock to his system—a reaction to stress that powered his imagination to positive action. Like some combat veterans, Russ could be moved to heroic duty to himself—a self-preservation move.

At another level, the rejection by Cheryl was only a temporary blow. It could have been more devastating, even to the point of motivating him to seek professional help, but it was offset by the access to mother. Mother had always "helped" and she would again, he believed. Mother, even at her best, could not do for him what he had to do for himself—battle the addiction dragon.

At yet another level, the rejection by society, which sent him to prison, gave him the opportunity to think about his behavior and he reacted by giving up drinking. His value system told him he had to conform, at least a little, to keep alive any hope for the life he silently yearned for—the life of his youthful idealism.

At Discovery House, he was confronted with his wished-for idealism and his current reality. They didn't match. Fortunately, his values were strong and solid. He had witnessed both parents claim competence in their world—they worked and shared their love of it with Russ early on.

Russ also witnessed their concern for quality—the determination value. The house was always in order, precious items were cared for, his parents persevered to make the family home comfortable. They showed a concern for nature and all that was within their world. He learned this lesson as well.

Family ties were established early. This teamwork display was further heightened by how father talked about his employees at work. Even one of Russ' early resentments about his father's going fishing with the boys later proved to be a broadening of the teamwork concept. At first Russ felt rejected because he couldn't go along. Today, he knows that his dad values his peers and treasures those friendships, a healthy and admirable trait, and an extension of the teamwork value.

Fran Latham communicated with Russ from childbirth. Her messages were usually positive and dynamic, helping him understand the value of dialogue. He misunderstood his father's stoic personality and took it as negative. Not until his father dropped his guard, and let his emotions out, did Russ realize the love that was there and how deep it really was.

In one sense, Russ is proving out Erikson's theoretical assumptions about cultural defiance, skills development, and stress management. A healthy sign is when a child's ideals come in conflict with his perception of the culture. Production occurs when the adolescent's skills are values-driven and based on what's learned in the fmaily. And it's both healthy and productive when external stress can be assimulated internally into positive behavior. In Russ' experience, it worked out well. He's turned things around.

In another sense, he's making an even stronger case for values development in early childhood. The values of the parents are built-in but their application, without guidance, may not be synchronous. This lesson can be replicated by other parents and teachers.

GUIDELINES ARE NECESSARY TO PRACTICING GOOD VALUES

If values are the triggers for appropriate behavior, then more parents will be less frustrated during their children's adolescent years if they practice more discipline. That doesn't necessarily mean punishment. Nor does it mean passivity. Discipline means consistent, fair, and immediate application of the core values. Here's an example of what one family's guidelines are and what it meant to its survival and growth.

- make clear what each family member's role is and what responsibility goes with it

- have a calendar of events for chores and fun, flexible enough to meet each member's needs
- resolve conflicts quickly as they occur, don't allow gripes or grievances to linger overnight
- make known the family traditions and abide and build on them as the years go by
- develop easy interaction amongst the family without stifling or putting anyone down with sarcasm
- be interested in each other's doings, share those experiences and learn from the outcomes
- develop a sense of unity by going out of your way for family members when the need arises without being a "patsy"
- play and have fun together to openly show love
- reach out beyond the family to neighbors and friends to broaden social and civic skills
- respect individual privacy and nurture individual differences especially as it applies to self worth
- listen to all the alternatives, make a decision and stick to it
- take the calculated risk to allow for the essential growth of each member within a spiritual climate.

These guidelines will serve the family well and develop individual skills needed for success in life. An adolescent who learns the core values and is given a chance to learn in the safety yet challenging home environment, where care and consideration dominate, will find that failure is not fatal.

These guidelines bear repeating because they develop the natural skills that Erikson and others discovered in their research on how people grow up. Notice the connections:

Clarity reduces confusion which leads to mistakes.

Achievement comes from a planned agenda of actions and events.

Industry is practiced when problems are solved as soon as they occur.

Integrity follows a path of systematic tradition and quality standards set at home.

Control need not be restrictive, but more of an interaction amongst supportive players who know the rules to follow.

Curiosity is developed by easy questions about one's experiences and answers obtained.

Trust is achieved by caring for one another and developing a natural bonding within the family.

Intimacy is gained without a smothering closeness as people play and honestly enjoy each other's company.

Generativity comes to be as people reach out to create a community of friends where new growth can take place outside the family.

Self Identity takes shape in private and develops within a nurturing environment of experimentation.

Autonomy is learned when everyone's wishes are heard and a decision is made in a win/win atmosphere, yielding to no excessive pressure.

Initiative is practiced by taking the calculated risk within the stretch beliefs that a Divine Power is with you.

A GAME PLAN FOR NEW PARENTS

Without these or similar guides, the new parent can be excited and threatened simultaneously by the responsibilities of the family. They had role models, their parents, and sometimes that was okay and in other cases it wasn't good enough. The role of parent is just not explained or laid out well in our culture. The injunctions for success are often mislaid, misspoken, or misunderstood without a game plan.

While the appearance at first glance, may be pedantic, the alternative, when it comes to alcohol and drug abuse, is harsh and objectionable. The mission is to keep children from senseless experimentation. The mission statement—the first part of the Parent's Game Plan (PGP)—should include words to the effect of using the family as a place for the adolescent to grow up. The crucial word in the mission statement is *"encouragement."*

A brief mission statement, then, would be:

"In order to build an acceptable living environment, we the parents will be encouraging of our children, allowing them to grow as individuals after entrusting them with our values through a series of lifelong role modeling."

DIFFERENT TYPES OF FAMILIES

Before getting into the next part of the PGP, which is an assessment of the child's (children's) potential, now is the time to look at different types of families and align with one or another. This appraisal is useful so the parents won't be saying one thing and doing another—like Tommy Ward's parents in the opening of each chapter.

Family Number One

In America, a large number of families conform to this specification: keep everything under control. They put their feelings, their beliefs and their intelligence aside at the first sign of crisis and put the lid down hard—keep it contained is the byword. There's no room for latitude, nor expression, nor relief. Keep it within the family, under control. Let no one else look in and see the dirty laundry, or offer assistance.

Family Number Two

A large number of families fit this second category and those are the ones who'll never give up. No matter how many times Johnny or Sally cheat or steal or weasel out of promises, they'll hang in there with all the familial wherewithal at their disposal. They are relentless in their hope. Anything else would be less than valid. The credibility of the family heritage is at stake and they'll never give up—even when they're broke.

Family Number Three

Close in description to Family Number Two, this family unit is destined to suffer, no matter what. They know it's their lot in life to bear the sins of their offspring. They have more than their share of guilt and they bear it out like the badge of courage it takes. Suffering brings out the best in them and they all wear similar hang-dog looks of despair. Suffering, you know, is good for the soul, or so they say.

Family Number Four

In some families, not too many fortunately, are the rescuers. When someone is in trouble, they take it upon themselves to get the victim out of the mess without making waves. They, like the Family Number One, will work to keep it together but one parent or the other generally takes the lead in doing all the work. They overlook a lot of symptoms and find it difficult in coming to grips with addictive behavior of their young.

Family Number Five

A small but growing number of families want the addict to get straight. They'll send him or her to this treatment or that and cross their fingers it'll work out. They won't do a lot of lifestyle changes, but they'll welcome some in their brood. In fact, they'll insist on it. The addict becomes a permanent part of the "closet" family if they don't conform. Grandparents in this family blame the parents if the children get in trouble.

Family Number Six

Another burgeoning group is the latest family type—learning from the experience. They may have acted too slowly but they did act. They sought help, for the addict first, and themselves next. They saw what went wrong, connected to it and set about to change what was necessary to strengthen the family tree. It hurt to trim some branches and cut some limbs, but in the long run the tree will flourish and grow straight.

Family Number Seven

This family will probably not experience the pangs of addiction because they already have a game plan in operation. All the players know the rules and they play hard with times to share the joys of winning and time out to rest from the effort. These are the lucky families who either had good role models or could adapt themselves if they didn't. They may have taken the time to listen to someone else's advice early on in the game. Pockets of these families are in America today. Not many, though.

Maybe a useful procedure would be to take a closer look at Family Number Seven to understand how they overcome some of the problems that confront all families.

THE CARING FAMILY

Parents that fall in this favorable category can't be statistically classified. Not that enough of these families aren't available for the sample but rather that they defy simple description. Some have college degrees, while others have street smarts. Some wear white collars, others blue. They are instinctive people—they know it's okay to teach their children about sexuality and self image.

Whether they knew it or not, these two aspects of growing up are the most common downfalls for adolescents. Sexuality or lack of understanding about it creates more anxieties and doubts about relating to others than anything else. Self image is a close second, and over the long term, is just as important in determining the prospects for success.

Caring, in this family, means literally taking care of the important things as they develop. When the baby boy plays with his penis, the parent doesn't panic. It's a natural act of exploration and not the cause for "naughty boy" messages. The same can be said for nudity. How the family handles nudity goes a long way in determining if the child grows up with a healthy respect for his or her body. Hardly anyone takes a bath or shower with clothes on, so nudity has an appropriate place in the household.

Family hugging and touching is a valid expression of care and love. Some people find it difficult to touch, and yet all the research shows it to be one of the most effective bonding acts of a healthy family. Eric Berne says stroke deprivation is one the leading cause of neuroses and psychoses in the world. The family that withholds strokes from its members is likely to experience a variety of difficulties. Early touching develops what Erikson describes as trust.

The caring family not only has guidelines, it has a system that is apparent to all its members. The system can be described, learned, and taught. It is factual; filled with spirited feelings and yet relaxed; it's visual; it's well-timed; and is based on real not perceived needs. In other words, it's a harmony that comes about because the parents pay attention to their own needs and those of the children.

This system is not always perfect—far from it. It's like a tight-wire act in the circus—it calls for good balancing. Sometimes it takes some real, hard work for the parent to not let expectations get in the way of real caring. Sometimes, it means the parent has to let go of reigns and allow the child to experience. Knowing when to keep control and when to let go is the problem. Too many parents hold on too long. A few let go too early.

The well-coordinated parent balances what they learned from their own parents with new logic and personal intuition. In Eric Berne's system of transactional analysis—the psychoanalytical treatment for out-of-balance people—the dogmatic or overly autocratic nature can be curbed with practice which means the dogmatic or overly authoritative nature of the person can be curbed through practice. With training, a true to life parent can be less domineering, especially under stressful situations. When this is achieved, the parent will function more reliably as a guide for the child, rather than an overly protective or permissive being.

The chances for successful child development flourish in an environment of structured experimentation. If only the parents could better confront the issues facing them and use them as grist for the mill. A recent parent/child survey conducted for use in this book indicated that five troubles loom large today. They are

1. the economy,

2. technology and change,

3. the information explosion which breeds insecurity and incompetence,

4. dual careers, and

5. the media.

GIVING UP THE RESPONSIBILITY

Parents, who are consciously or unconsciously troubled with these responsibilities infringing on how they are raising a family tend to turn over the duties to either the schools or television. *"I pay taxes and expect schools to educate my children so they'll be able to get jobs and participate in the community."* Or *"Sit there, Junior, and watch the cartoons, while I fix dinner, iron the clothes and talk with Mrs. Smith."*

The abdication is not viewed by them as a serious crime. But the end result is the same as if they abandoned the child in the nearest shopping mall. The schools are not prepared to function as character builders, nor is television even remotely close to its potential as an appropriate surrogate teacher.

H. Ross Perot, the multi-millionaire high tech wizard and social activist, claims that schools have become a little more than baby-sitters for America's young. He decided to do something about the lethargy in his home state despite cries from associates that nothing could be done. His work with the reform of the Texas public schools brought critical acclaim a few years ago, but the bureaucracy he uncovered is slowly regaining its position of eminent domain.

Perot changed the structure, and that was a monumental task, but he didn't get to the heart of the institution—the family.

Television, too, took on American society with a hail and hearty zeal. It was to be the greatest educational force the world has ever known. Something happened on the way to the forum, and it wasn't so funny. TV has not come close to its potential and as former Federal Communications Commission czar Newton Minow said, ". . . it's a vast wasteland." He said it 30 years ago and little has changed to remedy its status.

Since TV's inception in the late 1940s, it has popularized the family with *"Father Knows Best," "Ozzie and Harriet," "All in the Family," "The Jetsons," "The Flinstones,"* and recently with Bill Cosby as co-head of a dual career household, without a dint in the problem. Like radio before it and in the newspaper funnies, television has made buffoons of the characters in our hallowed institution.

Recent television programming and public affairs commercials have turned a serious focus on the drinking, drug, and cigarette problem in this country. It's gone from the early Sunday morning low viewership time slots to prime time almost overnight. Big name entertainers and sport celebrities now urge viewers to stop the insanity for the kids' sake. Even the beer advertisers call for driving-and-drinking safety.

Yet, the critical societal issues facing the family are glossed over in 30-second spots that point a finger without offering a hand. Violence in the family is epidemic. Divorce is rampant and only a last resort, which many are not able to take because of religious conviction. Drugs and alcohol are simple escape avenues for millions of troubled people.

Schools and television, however, will respond to mass public pressure. The job is to mount that campaign through small groups of interested parties. One national leader who says he wants to bring about such a coalition is former U. S. Senator Gary Hart. Hart, though, has a communications problem. He's a conceptual thinker (whole brained) and most of his audience is left-brained listeners.

If you look at what he says, rather than listening to him, you find yourself nodding your head in agreement. In fact, he's made quite a stir in Washington as a novelist. Hart's platform of a return to basic family values, service to country by young people, and ongoing education for a productive and competitive America makes sense.

NEOTENY AS A MODEL FOR FAMILY GROWTH

So much sense that it connects with anthropologist Buckminster Fuller who believes that the concept of **neoteny** will provide a valuable link missing in the family chain. Neoteny is the retaining of certain youthful characteristics into adulthood. By being zestful, energetic, and alert to opportunities, the family can regain its lost stature as a cornerstone of American society. The ingredients are openness, patience, dedication, and evaluation.

Openness, the first ingredient, is subdivided into several parts. Each family member makes an assessment of strengths and weaknesses based on left, right, and whole brain skills—a review of the Status Quo. (A questionnaire for this step is in Chapter 9. There's one for teens and one for adults—the results are the same.) This information is shared with each other without criticism, non-verbal put-downs (such as sighs, rolling of eyes, giggles or similar behavior), negative input or other than supportive commentary. What is is.

Another part of openness is to brainstorm issues that impact the family based on the five core values. For instance, economics. Parents may bring up how much money is available for allowances. Kids may indicate how much allowance they believe they need. On Determination, parents may indicate what constitutes a clean bedroom, clean bathroom, etc. Children may wish to develop a schedule for maintaining the quality of a clean house. On Teamwork, each member may put forth ideas for vacations, short trips, overnighters, etc.

The family list is built with no special emphases because of seniority, size, or similar factors. All input is considered valid and will be dealt with at a later stage in the process. No action takes place in the openness phase. A date and time is set for the second ingredient which is patience.

Patience is the brain's best friend. While the data from the openness phase sets to perculating in the mind, a phenomenon takes place known to some as insight and to others as Ah Ha—a connecting of disparate parts, a synergy. When the family gets back together—having spent some time allowing the brain to work on the data in its own spontaneous way—they discuss the outcomes of patience, i.e., insights.

Some insights involve dramatic changes of heart over where a vacation ought to be spent next summer. Often, one member makes a commitment to another member regarding one of the strengths or weaknesses (we prefer to call them areas for development; it's less negative). Or a question is asked to clarify something that was said or intended. The patience ingredient is merely an exchange of information based on the previous session. The next or third ingredient is, Dedication.

Dedication is the call to action. It's the application of one's energy used in the best rhythm possible. Not too intense, not too lax. Just right. Pads of scratch paper with plenty of sharp pencils also is required for this experience. This is not a win/lose game; it's trial and error experience. It's experiential, not academic. Like Einstein said, "play with the elements of the situation and see what develops."

One of the family issues is selected for discussion. It can be done so randomly or the item most strongly on the group's collective mind or by vote, whichever seems most feasible. Only one issue at a time. Once agreement on the issue has been forged then each writes about it in a stream of consciousness format. A favored writing technique of James Joyce, stream of consciousness is to write as much as possible, without stopping to think, analyze or edit. Four or five minutes is usually a good time frame.

Writers are encouraged to use symbols, numbers, words, images, colors, animals, phrases and so on, but not complete sentences. Stream of consciousness is not so much a literary, as it is an emotional experience. The outcomes of this writing generally produce a conceptual framework of the subject being examined. It may not be easy for some at first, but with practice, the ability to access what's on the mind becomes a lively and visual art.

THE 2/4/2 GAME

After quickly sharing verbally what was written, a game is played. The game is 2/4/2. It is played in teams of threes, if possible. If not, then in pairs. Or in some combination thereof. The lessons are learned best in the triad structure—a power of the pyramid configuration. It's best to allow an hour for this part of **Dedication.**

The rules are simple. Each member of the triad picks a skill that they want to develop—one skill from the survey in Chapter 9 (Figure 9.1). The member who begins the game then gives his or her views on the issue at hand, whether it's the vacation or clean bathrooms, and spends one minute going over the issue. The next step is to take another minute and talk about the skill just selected. Let's say it was problem solving. You describe how you use that skill today and what you would like it to be in the near future. Do that for another minute. One minute talking about the issue, another on the skill. Then, sit back and relax.

During your two-minutes of input, the other two family members were engaged in active listening. No talking to you, no questioning, just listening. Now they have an active role to play after your two minutes—they will discuss how you might use your problem solving skill to its best advantage on the issue at hand. They develop some options or strategies for you as if you weren't even there. They talk to one another without looking at you. You're relaxing and listening, remember? This goes on for four minutes.

Then you each write for two minutes about what you got out of the previous six minutes. You may want to do a stream of consciousness or merely jot some notes for two minutes. Do this in three rounds so that each person has a chance to input once, dialogue twice and write three times. At the end of the three rounds, you may want to share what you wrote with the other two and vice versa.

Keep at this until all the issues and all the skills have been addressed. It may take a couple of weeks. Don't rush. You will slip back and forth between Patience and Determination, but that's okay. You'll be developing a nice rhythm in the mean time.

When it's all done, a calendar is needed—one that's large enough to post on a wall or put on a flip chart. Magic markers, a different color for each member, is a good idea. Use the calendar as a guideposter. Someone, preferably someone with legible handwriting, is chosen to write the action steps on the calendar. Or each may want to use their own marker to post significant action steps.

It's a good idea to keep your own personal commitments on a separate calendar as well, but all family activities will be posted on the wall calendar. It will include skills practice, exercise times, nutrition hints, relaxation and quiet times, and so on. While it may appear to resemble gibberish at times, you'll know what it means.

The calendar is your scorecard, too. Figure out some creative way to mark the successes and near misses. There may be a few failures, but not enough to impede the process. You may want to set up an incentive system after a couple of months. Don't do that immediately until you've had some experience with the system and have had time to de-bug it. Incentives, once the program is understood by all and being practiced in good, spirited fellowship, can put a little more focus into projects.

WHAT IS NEOTENY

This program is designed for easy confrontation of real issues within the family. Take the easy ones first and become acclimated to working together. When the competencies and trust levels are in a secure place, then go after the more sensitive and troubling topics. Drugs, smoking, booze, ambitions, careers, choice of friends, hygiene, and so forth.

With the family in focus and working together, the chances are very good that adolescent experimentation will be healthy and vital. It may even rub off on the older members of the household. The fourth ingredient, evaluation, can be applied after you have applied the other three: openness, patience, and dedication.

SUMMARY

A family in crisis may be ready for constructive change. Like any change, it's best handled with care.

The caring family will establish some guidelines for optimal interaction. The content of the rules are often not as important as the process of getting them visualized, understood and acted out.

Erik Erikson has a way of connecting research to everyday living. Basic values of competence, determination, teamwork, communications and economics will drive a person to success. Individual skills are powered by these values in a positive, thoughtful way.

Staying youthful and filled with vitality is not as utopian as the "fountain of youth." It's more a matter of working at it together as a family.

CHAPTER 6

SESAME STREET REVISITED

Saturday mornings when most kids were up early mesmerized by cartoons on television, Tommy Ward watched the tube but concentrated on the documentaries and travelogues. For a 10-year-old, he showed a remarkable ability to comprehend adult themes, especially the adventurous aspects of life around the universe.

Ellen Ward wondered if Tommy would "miss out" by not being more of a child and take pleasure in the normal, fun things of being young. She wanted him to be less serious—her childhood had been so devoid of such simple pleasures.

"Tommy," she'd begin in a pleading voice, **"Are you sure you don't want to watch cartoons? They're so much fun, Honey,"** her voice trailing off, knowing the response before the words left her mouth.

"Shsh, Mom," he'd answer without looking at her, keeping a steady gaze at the screen, not wanting to miss a beat. His concentration was not like a boy nearing adolescence. He could block out anything when his mind was preoccupied with something of interest whether it be books, television or working on model ships—his favorite hobby. Often he kept a journal on programs he liked and had a stack of steno pads filled by the time he was ten.

His favorite stories—in books and on television—were of the sailors who roamed the seas, discovering new lands, and charting new courses. He would be aboard the Santa Maria with Columbus if wishes could be granted. Astronauts, too, took a lot of his attention. Tommy Ward was a born explorer.

TELEVISION AS A TEACHER

The trouble with television, say the critics, is that it has filled its programming time with unintelligent, action-packed and yet colorful drivel. Some say it's turning our children into moronic and stultified mirror images of what's seen on the screen. Research from leading universities indicates the brains of television-oriented youth are developing differently than the brains of those radio-oriented young people of yesteryear. **Different,** not better or worse. The research says we need more research, of course.

Without argument television makes a difference in how our culture is developing and, while the jury is still out on the good or bad of it, we continue to wonder where it will lead us. Too many parents, like Ellen Ward, are bystanders when it comes to viewing choice. Oh, we'll scream when it comes to sex and violence and draw the line there. But the violent themes of today's cartoons are as gruesome and undermining as adult shows on any given prime time evening.

Eric Hofer, the longshoreman philosopher, went so far as to say that the teen-age group in America has been expanded from the usual 12-to-19 age bracket to a larger, more encompassing 10-to-30 age range. Hofer believed television has given ten-year-olds the lifestyle of older juveniles while the post-sputnik education explosion keeps people on campus until their late twenties in a state of prolonged adolescence. A novel thought worth pursuing.

Hofer believed that children no longer exist. At least not the kind we used to be, and know. The public schools are packed with mini-adults hungering for the prerogatives of their elders. They want to be adults. They are bored with meaningless book learning and want action and skills associated with grown men and women.

Bored young people, we know, are disasters going someplace to happen. The adolescent, who has lost the child's capacity to concentrate and is without the inner resources of the mature, craves excitement and novelty to stave off boredom. Without these two characteristics—concentration and skills-adolescents become victim of their own devices. They work to exclude themselves from children and elders alike. Without wisdom and serenity, they'll take unnecessary risks—like getting intoxicated—to get what they think they want.

TURNING NEGATIVES INTO POSITIVES

Margaret Dowling of Oak Park, Illinois, near Chicago, is a risk taker. Married, the mother of three, Margaret is an entrepreneur. She left the comfort and security of work with a large candy manufacturer because "I wanted to do my own thing." Husband Terry was doing his thing in commercial real estate and they tried a couple of joint ventures, but still she felt tied down.

"I wanted to flap my own wings. My dad, who was my risk taking model, ran a service station in St. Louis and I wanted to run something. When the video tape recording business started to take off, I got aboard for the ride. It's been delicious!" she smiles as wide as the Mississippi. That's one side of it. The other side is pride in family.

"What I've learned as a new parent—and that goes for each addition in this family—is to stay close and watch these kids grow. Being my own boss, I can set my own hours. When any of my kids needs me, really needs me, I'm there. I love it. Watching them do something new for the first time is an experience I never want to forget. I fairly exploded with pride the first time Heather danced solo in ballet class. Or when Todd took off on his new bike. Or when Tyler built a house of blocks and it actually looked like a house...a real house with doors and windows and everything," Margaret bubbled.

Without going into a long story about it, suffice to say that things could have been different in their household. Margaret made a choice to teach her children values and skills. She knew enough about schools that it was a risk she didn't want to leave with the institution. Like Hofer, she knew that a few precious moments of childhood innocence can quickly pass and can turn into something less if you don't take the time to include these young people in your life at a very intimate and personal level.

In Figure 6.1 is a schematic diagram to describe how Margaret views this upbringing and uplifting experience and how others can do the same. The diagram details the Stages of Relationships and how each family can develop towards a synergistic unit.

Stage Five: SYNERGY

Stage Four: CONFIDENCE

Stage Three: AWAKENING

Stage Two: QUESTIONING

Stage One: STATUS QUO

Figure 6.1 Stages of relationships.

The first stage of any relationship is the **Status Quo.** It's a time to gather information in the safety and comfort of low pressure. The dialogue goes something like this:

> *"Is this your first time here?"*
>
> *"Yes, as a matter of fact, it is. Do you come here often?"*
>
> *"No, it's my first time, too. Can I buy you a drink?"*
>
> *"Yes, thanks, but I must tell you I'm expecting my boyfriend—he's a linebacker with the Bears."*
>
> *"Well, I'll see you around," he said picking up his change.*

So ends Stage One for this well-intentioned casanova. Had he been less faint-hearted and as skilled as Margaret Dowling in turning negatives into positives, he might have stayed around to meet a famous pro football player. That is if the young lady wasn't pulling his leg.

He didn't get to Stage Two which is **Questioning**—a place where you gather more data to affirm if you want the relationship to continue or not. The budding Lothario acted quickly and on only limited data. He lost what the future might have held for him because of his impatience. Stage Two is where you exchange information at a growing level of intensity. It could go like this:

> *"I see that you seem puzzled over which tie goes with that shirt. Can I help?"*
>
> *"Why yes you can. The blue tie matches the stripes, but the foulard catches all the colors, the stripes and solid shade. I can't make up my mind"*
>
> *"Well, most men have a solid blue tie hanging around somewhere. The foulard is a little dashing, though, and right now it seems to be the more stylish. I'd wear that one. Is it for your husband?"*
>
> *"No, it's for my Dad. A birthday gift."*
>
> *"Guess he's a Pisces, like me. Why don't we have a cup of coffee and talk over things astrological?"*
>
> *"Sure, I'm not into the zodiac all that much, but I have some questions about Pisces males. You might be more helpful than just selecting ties."*

By sticking to the subject and gradually expanding the scope of his questions, this adventurer moved right along. He took the opportunity on face value, moved the process further along with the probing question about who the tie was for, and capitalized on his good fortune when the answer opened the door for next moves. He moved them nearer the next stage, Awakening.

Awakening, Stage Three, is where a decision is made based on intellectual and emotional data to continue the relationship. Two things generally happen going from stage two to stage three. First, most of us don't ever get enough information to make a rational and logical decision, so we get stuck in the second stage. Or, we don't like being stuck so we make our choice on either logic or feelings—not a combination of both. You can write scenarios appropriate to either, I'm sure.

The key to reach stage three in the best shape is to take a risk—open up to both mental and emotional data involved in the situation. When the decision to move ahead is based on both logic and intuition, the chances of getting even further ahead are geometrically advanced. Without the balance, we enter Stage Four on one leg.

Stage Four is where ***Confidence*** is built as the two individuals experience more of each other over time. Let's look at an example:

> "Bill, come in here a minute. I want to go over this acquisition report on the Baxter deal."

As he walked to his boss's office, Bill wondered if all the t's had been crossed and the i's dotted. The boss was a bit of a nit picker. *"What's up, Lisa? Did I forget to tie it with a pretty pink ribbon?"*

"It's not a joking matter, Bill. I don't follow your assumptions about real estate values in that neighborhood. I can't submit this as it stands if you can't validate how prices are going to remain stable for three years when they haven't in the past 20. Can you make me feel more comfortable," Lisa looked him straight in the eye, sitting across from Bill in her open conference area.

"I'm playing a hunch, Lisa. I know it goes against the trends, but my gut tells me it's worth the risk. Sorry, I can't be more comforting for you."

> *"Well, Bill, I guess I'll have to shelve this proposal. I can't rely on any more of your gut shots. They haven't*

paid off yet. When you submit thoroughly prepared research, we get on with winning projects. I'm sorry, too."

Bill's spotty track record has a lot to do with Lisa's objections to his plan. She's in the Questioning stage in their relationship and so is he with her. He's skeptical of her ability, probably in part because she's female and in part because she's convinced that completed staff work means a balance between hard data and soft nuances. He has a tendency to skip over some of the factual facets and is, as yet, unable to match his intuitive side with hers. They'll keep vacillating from **Confidence** to **Questioning** until they overcome the skepticism they harbor for each other.

They'll not reach the top of the steps because **Synergy,** Stage Five, requires a complete melding of thinking and feeling. Few people reach and fewer still maintain this level in a relationship. Soldiers in combat units do. They rise to the top because their survival depends on complete trust in the other guys. School chums sometimes reach this peak because of a common, shared experience in a tough and intense situation. Women who have lived together in dorms and sorority houses tell of being able to regain that sense of synergy years afterwards in the snap of a finger.

Husbands and wives rarely reach this level and few children do with parents because they do not practice shared experiences enough. Going on picnics, or to the movies and so on simply is not finely focused enough to be an ultimate life experience. Most of what we have is a reaction to this stimulus or that. Synergy requires commitment and all-out participation from start to finish. It's not a hit-or-miss proposition.

This is the building block diagram that Margaret Dowling used in her relationships with those close to her. She didn't allow outside interests to keep her from doing what she decided years ago to do—raise a family, be her own boss and do both without loss of the other. Her relationship with husband Terry improves daily as they learn to be more open with each other. Doing so is not always easy nor painless, but it's moving in the right direction. Margaret knows that a negative in her life is an opportunity to turn that energy into something worthwhile. That's a mighty huge lesson she's learned.

THE ART OF INCLUSION

The late Dr. Gordon Lippitt of The George Washington University's school of behavioral sciences used to say that rejection was one of the most fear-producing events in a person's life. He couldn't imagine any other action that froze more people in their tracks. He believed that being shunned by another person created more anxiety than any other thing that could happen to a person. Rejection or the possibility of it is what keeps people on the second step of Stages of Relationships.

The other side of the rejection coin is *inclusion.* It's a fairly straight forward idea to grasp, although not as easy to implement. The best example of inclusion if the family—merely by being born into the unit are you included. No questions asked. Of course, when you do drugs, you risk exclusion. In the remaining situations, inclusion is often a dilemma.

Immigrants to this country have often faced a difficult task at being assimilated in the "melting pot." Blacks have felt the prejudice from a dominant white society. Women, trying to make equality a reality, took to the streets and tried vainly to legislatively correct a perceived injustice. New employees are confronted with cliques at work; students, the product of a mobile society, are new kids on the block and in school until they prove themselves. Labor had been outside of the mainstream until it gained enough power to offset Management. Aristocrats, intellectuals, militarists, priests, and even common people prize influence over other people—the power to reject or include.

Take Ben Litt, for instance. Ben earned a doctorate in the social sciences and was on the faculty at Lehigh University. His interests ran to why some people, more than others, were included or rejected. The included, he surmised, tended to have less problems with drugs, booze, and other substances, relying more on their own fortitude to survive the vicissitudes of life.

To further his research, he became part of a work/study program on power in the mid 70s. During the program, Ben experienced, for the first time, the emotional power of rejection and inclusion.

One of the exercises of the program called for each of the work groups to perform a series of tasks together to develop new skills and strengthen current ones. Over the course of time, the group became quite close—a bonding occurred, a natural inclusion, if you will. When the groups became solidified and loyalty was one of the more obvious characteristics, they were asked to exclude one member. This was a simulation similar to a situation at work where a reduction in force was prescribed.

Each group came up with a list of criteria on which to assess each member and, in essence, force rank the constituents. What it amounted to was a summary test of survival of the fittest. Because each member of the group was pre-selected for certain quality traits, no muffins were around. The task was formidable: Get rid of someone whom you've become quite attached to and do it in an orderly and thoughtful manner.

Dr. Litt was excluded from his group. For the next hour, he told of a disorientation he had never before experienced. He wandered around the familiar training grounds as though he had never seen the landmarks. When he came back to the group and wrote in his journal, he was feverish in his exposition.

The impact of this experience led him to drastically alter the way his work in education would continue. He restructured his academic leanings to experiential methods. He quit lecturing to his students, telling them about theories and concepts. He allowed his students to learn by doing and then recording what they thought and felt about the experience. Just like he did following his exclusion. And just like Tommy Ward did when watching something important on television.

The first step in inclusion, Dr. Litt discovered, was to get in touch with thoughts and feelings and the best way for that to happen is to access what's going on in your mind and body. Accessing the great storehouse in your brain is done by journal writing.

Earlier described, keeping a journal is one facet of the explorer. Columbus, Magellan, Cortez, the astronauts, and other great world and space adventurers kept track of their journey by keeping a written record. Some kept a separate log to maintain a memory of rational events in a timely manner and a journal to recall their impressions and feelings, a more spontaneous and intuitive writing.

Dr. Litt read aloud from his journal to his group. Even those who had felt exclusion on a different level at a different place could not relate to Ben's devastation. Here was a man with impressive credentials, a maturity earned through hard knocks, and the ability to articulate at several levels, and yet he couldn't handle exclusion. Those in power were somehow immunized from his hurt and discomfort. They could not empathize.

Later, when the inclusion exercise had been completed, the other members realized how they had been part of the hurt-Ben process. They found out that people in power frequently don't act as sensitively as they do when sharing power. They make assumptions about people they know, which often don't work out. The idiom that power tends to corrupt and total power corrupts completely couldn't have made better sense to that group, in retrospect. An analogy can be made that parents have complete power and in turn are insensitive to their family's needs often to the point of exclusion.

ACCESSING ENERGY

Ben Litt regained his equilibrium and found new strength as the result of new learning. He found it through the search for better ways of learning. Dr. Litt knows that the **schools are producing learned but not learning people. Inclusion, he says, is the source of energy.** This does not mean joining every club or group that proffers entrance. Nor does it mean wanting to be part of all segments of society. It means being included in those that you need for self-sufficiency.

You may get a temporary high—like snorting coke—when the country club takes you in as a member, on a provisional basis, of course. You may or may not really need that membership to make you a better person. In most cases, it's irrelevant. Temporary highs are nice, but not necessary.

Necessary is what's critical here.

Through accessing your whole brain, you'll develop your ability to visualize. **Visualization is the path to power.** If you look at how most people dissipate their energy, you'll see why visualization is so crucial:

> inner struggles,
>
> self indulgence,
>
> incessant talking,
>
> reacting to pressure,
>
> game playing, and
>
> victim association.

Inner Struggles

Half of all the problems we face today, which consume an inordinate amount of our energy and time, are contained within us. Should I take the promotion and be forced to move again? Will he not drink so much tonight or will it be one argument after another? We have the ability to stymie ourselves in action by turning things over in our minds until we have exhausted the most productive parts of our selves. We can be more useful by making decisions sooner and with greater conviction. You simply do it, using all the information now at hand.

Self Indulgence

Another costly energy-sapping behavior is self indulgence—the worst way of feeling sorry for yourself. People stuck on the second level of Stages of Relationship, questioning, are usually self-indulgent because they do a lot of questioning of others without taking responsibility for learning the answers themselves.

For instance, Kitty Price was a school teacher who wanted to do more. She didn't quite know more of what, but knew that teaching didn't suit her. Or least it didn't seem to because she was restless. Her marriage foundered, and though she loved and adored her only child, she searched frantically for the right path to follow. Her frenetic behavior took her down many wrong roads. She indulged herself by constantly asking others for the answer to questions about life and its purpose. She couldn't quiet herself long enough to look inside and see the light. Her relentless pursuit of the wispy substance of life tired her and she was frequently drained and had this ill or that.

When she learned to quiet herself and look inside, she discovered basic and simple answers.

Incessant Talking

The incessant talker is an energy spoiler. These are the guys and gals when you ask the time of day will tell you how to make a watch. They generally suffer from an inferiority complex and are insistent on overcoming it right there in front of you. They not only tire themselves out, although you rarely see them without lips flapping, they wear out all others within ear shot. What they need to practice is the practical art of listening and getting in touch with feelings.

Reacting To Pressure

When you push a certain button on Willy Curtins, he jumps through a varied assortment of hoops. Willy is the nervous type and susceptible to external pressure of every sort. Reactive, Willy doesn't have a plan although he's a very good problem solver. He's a tactician without a strategic overview. Pressure gets to Willy and so does stress. He's frequently down with colds, the flu, sinus trouble, back aches, and the general feebles.

When Willy began to order his life around a plan, his symptoms disappeared and he took command of the wild swings of stressful situations. He took his skills, put them into a system and reacted less to the threat of doom and more to the opportunity they offered.

Game Playing

Psychotherapist Eric Berne noted that game players are abundant in American society—they fall into a broad range of types and Berne wrote a book about the most frequently played psychological games and the adverse effects you can expect from them. Like a good author, he also told how to curb the devastation from them.

Games, to Dr. Berne's way of looking at them, are a crooked way of living life. A game like "If It Weren't for You," a favored one of spouses, allows the players to waste time and energy over a wide range of issues. IWFY allows one person to "blame" another for not doing something the first one was afraid to do in the first place.

Mildred Farnham had a childhood phobic fear of becoming an alcoholic—both of her parents drank to excess. Her husband, Hy, kept her from socializing, and thus running the risk of drinking, because he was an outdoorsman and they spent all free time in the woods and mountains. She belly-ached about her restricted social role with neighbors and friends. Fights between Mildred and her husband led to his feeling guilty and brought her gifts to make-up. This game kept them from being intimate and the resulting sexual dysfunction caused less than joy in the marriage.

When they had professional help in looking at their lives, they confronted the game, overcame her fears, reduced his dominance and expanded their social life to the degree that proved acceptable and healthy to both.

IWFY is a game, too, that works in the same destructive way for parents with children. A child may have a fear of this or that and the parent keeps from confronting that fear but damaging the relationship in the process. They spend a lot of energy as they argue and make-up but never appropriately proceed to a healthy state of intimacy.

Victim Association

So it seems that birds of a feather do flock together. A victim of one game will associate with other like victims. The coffee-klatsch features all the wives of domineering husbands. The locker room harbors the guys sitting around playing "Yes, But," games that preclude problem solving any issue because the victims don't want the problem solved, they want the attention of other players. These and other illicit forms of taking energy away from productive use are universal in America homes and at work.

Sticking together is the framework for peer pressure and allows a convenient cover for those unwilling or unable to take the risk of responsibility for their own convictions and actions. Alliances are fine when the members know the objectives and the rules of the road. Otherwise, it's a con and debilitating.

The way out is to build a support network that includes a diverse-enough composition of personalities that allows for clean analysis of thinking and feeling. A mentor, too, is a necessary component for healthy relationships. A dutch uncle should be part of everyone's family situation.

THE WISDOM AND SERENITY MODEL

One of the treasured and underused words in the American lexicon is **perspective.** Thousands of parents wish their offspring had it. Adolescents wish their parents had it. Employers would ransom their cash flow for a clearer perspective. The artist thrives on it. The dictionary says it's a mental and true view of things in relative importance to each other—a visual prospect of reality.

To make our energy work for us—to keep it in perspective—we need a model, or a structure to build relationships with our significant others. **Wisdom** and **serenity** are the keys to this model. **Wisdom: the accumulated good sense, judgment, and philosophic and scientific knowledge. Serenity: a calm and unruffled involvement—a nonattachment to the dynamics of life.** Together, wisdom and serenity, can develop the synergy necessary for living to be a healthy 120 years old.

Some react to that statement like it was shot right out of a gun aimed at their temple. *"Who wants to be that old?"* Or,

"What kind of world would we have with all those old people in it?" Others, however, tilt their heads, smile, and think long and hard about the prospect. Imagine, 120 years old and relatively healthy.

A review of the medical and scientific information currently available to us, the possibility is there. The probability is not. It would require a discipline we aren't currently accustomed to and not likely to engender immediately. But we could if we really wanted it.

We'd need a great incentive. Like, say, a drug-free culture for our children to grow up in and live full, healthy lives.

Given an incentive that would create a reordering of personal and professional priorities, the wisdom and serenity model would fit. We need a guideline to follow, a pattern to test our efforts against.

Wisdom

First, wisdom. Alcoholics have a version that goes something like this: give me the courage to change what needs to be changed, the perception to know what can't be changed and the wisdom to know the difference. Wisdom also means pushing the limits a little further than they currently are.

Wisdom involves developing a discipline to learn new skills and create new interests. Not so you can be everything to everybody, but rather to be more of a renaissance man or woman—multi-talented, instead of single-minded.

Wisdom also means having philosophy of life. Too many Americans miss out on much of their own culture because they stick too close to it. They've little to compare. By shutting out other than their own singular entity, much excitement is shadowed. They fail to listen to the other guy's argument and so don't learn more about an issue. Truth is the whole. Sometimes that isn't pleasant and means we have to give up a prejudice to see it. Wisdom comes from truth and is mainly a left-brained experience although not necessarily limited to that hemisphere.

Serenity

Serenity on the other hand is probably more difficult to attain. It means playing the game within limits. Just as wisdom means pushing the limits, serenity calls for acceptance of the playing field as is. It's the practice of patience. Yet, it's not giving up. Being serene is being assured that what's happening is for the best as long as you were wise in planning. Serenity is the ebb and flow of nature in it's ultimate harmony.

We have to experience serenity to know it. Because it's mainly a right-brained phenomenon, the feelings associated with this reality are generally not easily recognizable to many of us. We have grown up in a culture that is dominated by Type A behaviors—rapid-paced, aggressive, loud and impatient—while almost the opposite can be said of traits of serenity. Calm in the face of pressure and stress, inscrutable in conflict, peaceful without being passive, and so forth.

Whether serenity can come without wisdom is arguable. Like the chicken and egg controversy, they are intertwined—related to the point of need. Together they provide us with a new dimension of ourselves, a higher order of understanding and purpose. The synergy of these two important human goals results in the most powerful condition possible. Wisdom is impersonal, while serenity is a more personal quality—the content and process of life.

Without serenity, wisdom is like a gadfly, bouncing from pillar to post with incessant chattering. No one listens. Conversely, without wisdom, a person who is serene is thought of as a vegetating being—not dynamic, not relating to issues and opportunities, a bear hibernating in the dead of winter. This model of living is needed to be all we can be.

While information doubled every twenty years in the 1950s, it's doubling at the rate of every five years or less today. Without a model of life, we're likely to fall victim of not knowing or being overcome by the pressure of trying to keep up.

BLUNDERERS, MADMEN, AND OTHER FEEBLE ATTEMPTS

Dick Carlson thought of himself as a sophisticate living in Portland, Oregon. He worked hard, earned a substantial salary, had gone to good schools, was a risk-taker, and generally was seen as a well-rounded individual. Wise, maybe; serene, he wasn't.

Dining with his college-sophomore daughter and a friend one night, the subject of drugs came up and Dick, as an informed parent, lashed out at the schools and government for not taking more of a stand on the spreading disease. He said that children from good homes would not go around ingesting substances that could cause serious injury and even death. He pointed to Stanford, where his daughter studied, as a prime example of a drug-free campus because of the high calibre of the students, faculty and the society from which both came. *"Why, I'll bet they don't even use marijuana there anymore,"* he offered.

The friend turned to the daughter and said, *"Tell him the facts of life."* She hesitated only a moment and then laid out a scenario that can be seen on virtually every campus in this country. Many of the kids smoke dope, most drink booze and although not too common, hard drugs are available and used. Most are used in combination and with cigarettes. While on the wan, they still are used to blow away anxieties.

She couldn't explain what "too common" meant. No one pressed her as to her habits. Dick Carlson, mouth ajar, learned that a certain percentage of young adults (Hofer's "adolescents") run the risk of addiction every day as a part of their need to be different than their parents.

The friend made the point that parents, as a class of people, simply were not up to date on what their children were up to whether as the most expensive schools or the state-supported colleges. Dick Carlson went quietly and thoughtfully for the rest of the evening. Hard to tell whether he learned anything or was miffed because he was made to look bad in front of his favorite offspring.

SUMMARY

Proud parents lose some knack as their children grow and they don't communicate as once they did. The pride can be turned on again if they really tried.

Learning the Stages of Relationships is an essential part of the communications at several levels cycle. People who are stuck and indulgent tend to only reach the second step and stay there.

People who are rejected need to find ways for inclusion. The most normal place for taking care of that is at home. Work is another good place to practice.

Keeping a journal is an approved way of exercising your whole brain. Explorers learned long ago that recording your thoughts and impressions goes a long way to insure personal growth and joy.

Adolescence, a period that Eric Hofer believes has an extended life today, requires more parental attention as well as experiential skills development—hands-on learning, they call it.

CHAPTER 7

SIGNS OF THE TIMES

The dice hit the wall and spun around until a voice yelled out, **"Seven, you lose."** The youngster who yelled scooped up the dollar and change, took the dice and said, **"Two dollars open. Who's crazy enough to cover me?"**

While the crowd in the garage bickered and pushed and made side bets, one of the players asked Tommy Ward if he had a cigarette. **"No, I don't smoke."** The return look and remark, **"What good are you,"** made Tommy wince. The garage was his cousin's and all the older boys seemed deeply engaged in the crap game and no one noticed how Tommy looked or felt.

He tapped the player on the shoulder and said, **"I know where I can get some."** **"Yeh? Well, go get 'em, Runt,"** the player shrugged him off.

Tommy ran the few blocks to his house where he knew his father kept a carton of smokes in his top dresser drawer. While running he thought that by getting the pack, he'd become part of the older group of boys, who seemed to not take much notice of him.

His father was out of town and his mother worked out back in the garden and he went directly to their bedroom. Tommy had never taken anything from their bedroom before and the thought hit him: Was this stealing? **"Well, maybe, but it's only a pack of smokes and Dad'll never miss one pack. Besides, I can make it up to him some other way,"** he reasoned and the conflict was resolved.

Opening the drawer, he found the carton with six or seven packs in it—that's great, he'll not miss one with so many left—took one and was about to close the drawer, when he noticed the revolver in the holster at the back.

The gun had a shiny metal finish and a pearl-handle. He had never seen it before and was tempted to take it out and look at it. But he was in a hurry so he merely pressed the trigger...

BOOM!

The bullet went through the one drawer, then another, hit a metal file cabinet in the corner and ricocheted back, nicking Tommy's head just above the ear. As the room filled with smoke, the nine-year-old youngster shook shakily, stunned by the noise, blood starting in a little trickle down his face.

That's how his mother found him when she screamed, **"My God, Tommy. What happened?"**

"I was looking for Dad's swim trunks," *he lied, setting up a more plausible argument in his mind for the later confrontation.*

NEED FOR CONFLICT RESOLUTION SKILLS

Conflicts in adolescence are an inevitable part of the growing up process. All people face inner conflicts—the kind stemming from emotional and intellectual aspects of their personality—and external conflicts, those which come from people and events confronting them in this situation or that. Adolescents rarely have the skills to deal well with either, although they probably seem to get by better with external ones.

In Tommy Ward's case, he flunked in both aspects. He reacted to the pressure from the older boy who asked for the cigarette. Instead of letting it drop after saying he didn't smoke, he felt the pressure to do something. So he ran home after a pack of cigarettes.

Once home, he felt the inner conflict: Was this stealing? Of course it was and he knew it. But the first conflict still had not been resolved and he found himself and his value system in a vulnerable condition. Confronted with another conflict—bam bam—Tommy became overstressed and disoriented. So he did what most other adolescents would do—quickly rid himself of the inner problem with a rationalization—Dad will never miss one pack.

The energy to complete the theft was made easier when he saw that the carton contained many packs. Had there been only one or two packs, it may have caused another stressful conflict for Tommy.

Even so, he was beleaguered by dual conflicts. Tommy probably would not have pulled the trigger on the revolver, causing another dire consequence, had he not been overloaded with conflict. He was, in normal situations, a thoughtful and respectful young boy. Under the stress of trying to be too much, too soon, he fell victim to stress and strain—a child's inability to resolve conflicts in a rational and emotionally balanced way.

Ask any normal parent what they would have done in a similar situation and you'll receive a wide range of answers—hardly any of which would have **processed** the event with the youngster. Hardly any parent would have helped him understand what triggered his need to steal, the need to pull the trigger, the need to lie. The trouble is that helping someone learn from a mistake is not viewed as high on our list of priorities. We didn't learn that way and how can you expect parents to teach their children in such a manner.

One reason that so few parents can **process,** in part, is because so few are professional conflict resolvers. Oh, they may be at work, but few have mastered it within the confines of the family structure. A skill at work is often left there. It's as if utilizing at home an affective ability learned at work is stealing from the employer. And what a waste of talent that really is. Because utilizing conflict resolution skills is needed to help overcome substance abuse. Conflict resolution is a critical skill to keep kids off drugs. Parents and children alike must come to terms with conflict in a smooth and satisfactory system.

TEACHING AND LAW ENFORCEMENT: COMPANIONS?

Nearly 20 years ago, the concept of "Officer Friendly" was devised in Concord, California by a low-ranking police officer, who had schools as his beat. The cop had a number of alternatives facing him. He could have slammed a program together, walked away from it and said, *"There, that's done."* Or he could have turned it back to the schools and asked them what they wanted and it would have become another bureaucratic committee, studying and studying what it wanted.

What he did, though, was look at the situation as a conflict between two institutional bodies—schools and law enforcement. Because he happened to be a cop in uniform with a teacher's heart, the Officer Friendly program became a valuable one in helping youngsters learn some fundamental rules of social safety. The program has since been copied and emulated by communities across the country with Godspeed and assistance from the Concord PD.

The die, it seems, has been cast in Concord. The cop who gets the school beat, inherits the institutional conflict. This time around, however, the conflict has been expanded to include substance abuse. Oh, Officer Friendly had that on his agenda, 20 years ago, but the new guy on the beat wants to do something about preventing the problem instead of reacting to it. He's a conflict resolver.

David Nye is 33 years old, a big man, not as rough and tumble as you might expect with boundless energy. Type A behavior would be a quick but inaccurate description. He's more a metallurgist with a ball-peen hammer, scientifically pounding metal into new and more durable shapes.

Those who really know him realize that David does take on hard things, but with finesse, a new police skill. Like his predecessor, Officer Nye is a teacher, not a stereotypical cop. His bent is talking and listening and his audience is young people. *"They were upset at first when I asked second and third graders to help edit a new version of a safety workbook."*

"They said I was supposed to 'tell them' what to do. When the project was finished, they knew that the give and take meant more than a lecture would have," he said, explaining his style.

David practices the Pygmalion Concept—if you see positive, you get positive—and he sees a lot of good in today's elementary school children. Unlike most police and law enforcement officials, David sees the brighter side of life. This adds to his already powerful source of energy. As a former beat and patrol officer, he knows the other side equally well and wonders how and when the conflict can be resolved given current policies, procedures, and attitudes.

"I'm on a task force with local educators and we're working on a full-scale approach to substance abuse. We're looking at next Fall to begin a new effort at education. I can't honestly say what it will contain or how we'll get it across, but I get the sense that it will be different than what's currently being offered. That sure hasn't worked, so we have to be risk-takers and be more creative," David added.

That may not sound like much, but coming from a cop, it has to take some by surprise. David comes by it naturally. He's not exactly a revolutionist but is creative.

His background is steeped in old fashioned American values, including the idea of service. His brother is a teacher and his sister a nurse. A major part of David's education was the good fortune of sharing a room for five years with his paternal grandfather at the onset of adolescence. While some young people would object, especially at that age, to giving up the prospect of a private room, David welcomed the opportunity.

He knew what fun would come from spending many hours with the man who had been so much a part of his happy, early years. What he didn't bargain on was seeing the other side of old age. The side that comes with poor health and despair. This experience of viewing the deterioration that unfortunately often accompanies the aging process gave young David a basis for conflict resolution that stands him in good stead today.

The Greeks, who seemed to have a word for almost every event or situation, expressed great regard for utility—using all effort and experience to its best advantage. David took advantage of his five years with Grandpa Nye as a means to greater understanding of life's process. The oldest law of nature being the cycle of birth-growth-death. Insights into the cyclical flow keeps him tracking with ways to change and implement child development.

NEW WAYS OF MANAGING CONFLICT

Rensis and Jane Gibson Likert of Hawaii wrote a powerful dissertation of "New Ways of Managing Conflict" several years ago in which they spelled out a supportive system for use in a variety of societal and organizational situations. Its major lesson is that most external conflict can be managed, not necessarily resolved.

Some problems, they argue, just can't be resolved satisfactorily so the next best thing is to keep them under some kind of control, i.e., labor and management strife, U.S. and Soviet relations, etc.

The Likerts discuss the conflict in schools, cities, corporations, and the like and describe how their system applies in each case. Although they don't take on the parent/child controversy, their system, with minor adaptation, can be predictive of major gains in these conflictful relationships. An easy procedure would be to overlay the Likert approach to five categories of parent/children conflict. The graph (Figure 7.1) helps describe them.

The five categories are represented by positions in Figure 7.1. In the lower left is where conflict is ignored and nothing is said nor listened about it—a lose-lose situation. In the upper left is where all listening occurs with no dialogue or plans for action—a likely win-lose prospect. In the middle of the figure is where some talk and some listening occurs but to no great degree or level of satisfaction—another lose-lose predicament. In the lower right is where extensive talk by both parties and little or no listening occur—a win-lose possibility. In the upper right where the epitome of the art of listening and talk ratio occurs, where enough time is taken to gather all the data and develop reasonable action from it—a win-win situation.

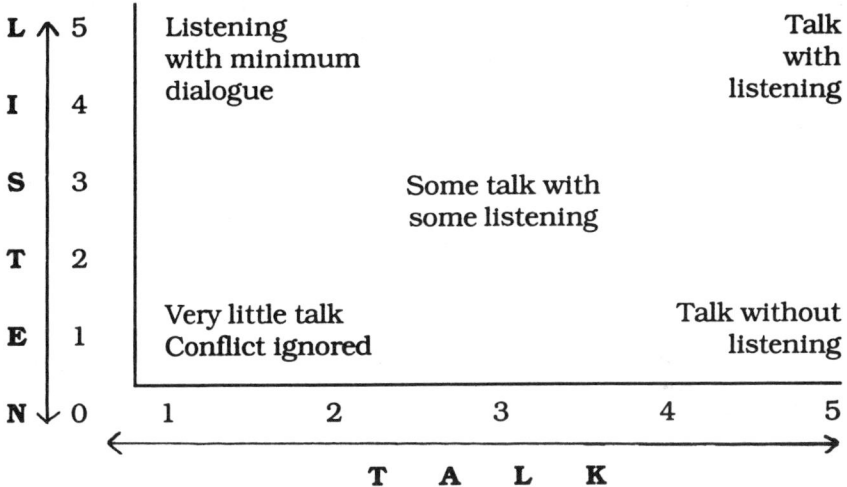

Figure 7.1. A parent-child discussion model.

Going from a win-lose or a lose-lose orientation, which has been the major conflict resolution model in this country's history, to a win-win possibility has a growing number of supporters even amongst lawyers who have been most notorious in preserving the traditional approach. Win-win precludes compromise—in fact it insists on it. And, if you change the motivation from compromise to collaboration, you make inroads at a faster and more predictable rate, moving to the upper right hand sector.

Collaboration means that you bring all interested and involved parties into the process as early as is possible. Like David Nye did with the elementary school children. When people are a part of the solution, they're less apt to be part of the ongoing problem.

Collaboration is David Nye's secret weapon. He holsters it in his work with addicts and in the prevention of addiction. When a criminal decides to reform and go straight, Nye will listen. When a teacher asks for help in the classroom, Nye gives it.

When other officers inquire about openings in school and drug prevention, he welcomes their questions and considers their assistance.

For instance, the proportion of listen/talk ratio is a learnable trait. Any issue that troubles a family, a married couple, a parent and teacher, or any two people or groups in conflict can be brought closer to agreement by learning observation skills. The key is to bring in a third party to practice observer techniques. Two people take opposite sides of issue while the third person observes the process. Here's the format for three people to follow:

1. Each makes a non-emotional statement about his or her perspective of the issue.

2. Both parties have a prescribed amount of time to ask for clarification and definition of terms used, one after another.

3. Each is asked to re-state the other's point of view.

4. A dialogue—each party has to spend equal time talking and listening—is held for a brief time with the intention of reaching agreement.

5. An observer reports to both on the process—who was aggressive, resilient, resistive, collaborative/competitive, etc.

The use of a third-party, interested but non-biased observer can often bring clarity to the scene, especially because adults with an emotional perspective miss out on the process of a discussion. After a little bit of experience as an observer, the contestants can incorporate observation into their debate and increase the likelihood of conflict resolution. Without being able to observe the process, bias reigns.

This skill is sometimes totally absent when you see frenetic and aggressive participants shouting and wailing away at each other. The prospect of agreement is unlikely and nothing is gained except reassurance that "I was right in the first place," or being lower right on the resolution scale—talk, talk, talk.

THE POWER OF CONCENTRATION

Golfer Jack Nicklaus, when winning more golf tournaments than other professionals before him, had the ability to shut out every distraction and focus completely on each shot on the course. You can still see him line up a 20-foot putt in sections—looking first a few feet ahead, then a few more and finally the last few feet into the cup. He imprints these sections in his mind and then uses the needed energy in the stroke to guide the ball into the hole. That's concentration, the key to conflict resolution.

Like Nicklaus, other athletes—basketball players stepping to the free throw line, baseball players stepping into the batter's box all make a practice motion to get the desired movement fixed in their mind before performing the act live. Better performers know that immediate rehearsal is critical to keeping themselves in focus—shutting out other distractions and keeping their entire physical, mental, and emotional selves fixed to the task at hand—all senses working in harmony for achievement.

Not many other professionals do this simple task of preparation. Most of us allow distractions and interruptions to throw us off our game. Getting in focus in business, school, or at home is as essential as it is on the playing field. Listening requires concentration. So does talking. Both are most relevant when they have been positioned to be inclusive—geared to success.

The most recent research on concentration stems from stress management work, mainly that of Dr. Meyer Friedman, who associates stress and its debilitating after effects with lack of concentration. Strange as it seems, concentration is a stress-related, personal activity. Too little stress results in weak or less than optimal concentration. Too much results in tiring and damaging concentration. The appropriate amount of stress in a situation for a given person results in optimal concentration and focus. For sake of this description, regard concentration and focus as the same with stress being the parallel aspect of it.

Friedman finds that excessive stress, that most often associated with Type A behavior, causes cardiac, gastro-intestinal and related disease—even cancer has been linked to stress. Suffice to say that stress in its aberrant form is not welcome. Researchers also tells us that a certain amount of stress is necessary to function in any society and that individuals vary in their susceptibility to adverse reactions to stress. One man's meat is another man's poison seems to fit the description of the variance of stress and its impact.

Researcher, Dr. John Adams of Washington, D.C., believes that stress is cumulative and that the body stores the excesses somewhere on muscle and organ tissue, developing a kind of body armor. Unless this stress-produced armor is taken care of by periodic and total release, the subsequent illnesses described by Mike Friedman can and do occur.

Millions of Americans treat their stress symptoms regularly through exercise, relaxation, proper nutrition, and support networks. Exercise rids the body of accumulated tensions, relaxation helps keep the bodily system loose and flexible. Nutrition enables the body to sustain prolonged periods of stress abuse and to renew stress damage along with rest and exercise. Support groups provide a release for some tensions that are more psychological and not easily handled by simple exercise, diet, and relaxation. Dr. Adams and others insist that a complete stress management program include all four components.

What most Americans, however, do not do is abstain from stressful situations, events, and people. Some times we can't. Our job may require us to continually confront a boss or subordinate, a customer or a spouse that creates unharmonious conditions. We may be able to withstand these conditions for a certain length of time, but inevitably the banging that stress does on our body and psyche shows damage. This damage is similar to the damage that drug, cigarettes, and alcohol abuse manifests.

STRESS AND CONCENTRATION RELATIONSHIP

One of the first symptoms of stress abuse is loss of concentration. We can't seem to keep our minds on the subject.

Our rational skills get fuzzy and we tend to wander off easily. As with the chicken and egg controversy, which comes first, stress or concentration? Stop-gap methods to improve concentration are in reality stress management techniques so how you approach the problem really doesn't matter—both can be attended simultaneously and with similar results.

All of the stress management and concentration tricks are coping mechanisms—they do nothing to relieve the source of the stress. Exercise, diet, relaxation, and networking regimes are useful and necessary health attributes but they don't get the monkey off our backs.

> **Activity.** One of the in-the-meantime methods of temporarily regaining the strength of concentration is by a combination of physical, mental, and emotional exercises. You can stand, sit, or lie down. Be in a place where you'll not be interrupted for at least 10 minutes. Have the secretary hold the phone, lock the bedroom door, whatever. Start with deep breathing. Inhale deeply through the nose, if possible, and release slowly through pursed lips. Release your breath from the bottom of the diaphram up through the lungs to the mouth. Imagine a flexible tube going from the pit of the diaphram to your mouth.
>
> Think only about your breathing, ridding your mind of extraneous thoughts. After eight or ten deep breaths, you'll be calmer than when you started. Close your eyes and imagine yourself outdoors in your own backyard. Notice the surroundings, the sounds, the colors. Imagine yourself rising above this area to a height of 18 or 20 feet. Turn yourself around so you are looking down at the area. Notice how it now looks . . . the colors . . . the sounds. Turn yourself around, so you're looking at the blue sky and white clouds.
>
> Elevate yourself up into the clouds, feel the milkiness and coolness of the clouds, come out and face upward until all you see are the blue clouds. Feel the freedom. Turn yourself around until you are facing the white, billowy clouds. Find an opening in the clouds. Go to the opening and come back down to earth to a place where you had a recent, pleasant experience. Relive that recent pleasant experience.

After three minutes (set an alarm clock or wrist alarm) return to where you are now, open your eyes at your own discretion and pace. Notice how you feel physically, mentally, and emotionally. If you can, share the experience with someone near you or write your thoughts and feelings in your journal.

Following this meditative experience, most people are less stressed and able to better concentrate on what lies ahead. This is especially useful for when confronting conflict. For example, if all the members of the family went through this activity as a preliminary step to a family conference, it might well expedite the outcomes. The outcomes would be favorably enhanced if the sharing part became a preamble to actual issues development and confrontation.

Being in a state of "soft focus" as compared to "hard focus" is useful to creative and high performance. Soft focus enables you to be relaxed, yet alert, ready to work in a more harmonious condition. Staying in soft focus is a desired state of well being. Former tennis professional and Davis Cup coach Arthur Ashe calls it being in the "zone." Professional athletes of all sorts have remarked on the state and described the feeling from "playing inside yourself" to a "can't miss" situation.

Other drills and activities are available to attain this state, but none are likely to last as long as you continue to face unchanged stress conditions in your life. Another ingredient to be examined and acted upon is **time**—the most wasted and important aspect of creative living.

TIME WAITS FOR NO ONE

Earlier, author Eric Berne's idea of how we spend time was described and can now be elaborated. Berne felt that Americans, most noticeably, have a great need to structure time even though we are notorious for misusing the moments at our disposal. After cookbooks and diet programs, the most sought after books in this country are on time management. Numerous courses, offering hints on how to handle the hours at work, and consultative workshops and seminars abound on the subject. Calendars of endless variation on slotting activities into color-coded, A, B, C priorities can be obtained at any bookstore, office supply, and related retail outlet.

The truth is that time is not the issue, of course. We agonize over how slow it goes, how fast it goes, how we can't get enough of it, how it sits on our hands, and so forth. We have come to blame it for a host of personal and societal ills. The reality is that time has become the scapegoat for more serious and deadly sins. It boils down to a lack of philosophy and a plan to live accordingly.

Yet, some of us manage to accomplish a great deal in spite of time constraints. Those who resist time-robbers with the best accommodation are the professionals in their chosen work. They know that the telephone can be hazardous to your health and have a system to screen callers. They also spend three minutes or less on many calls because they plan ahead. Research tells us that too many people at work spend eight to ten minutes on a three-minute call. Even without research on social calls, one can deduct from visible evidence that excessive time is spent on obtaining minimal information especially in homes where teenagers actually use the telephone as an extension of the schoolyard or soda shoppe.

A part of the problem is we don't know how to say goodbye—a misplaced belief is that cutting off a phone conversation is discourteous or impolite—and another part is that we don't have a conclusion in mind before we call. Berne would call this latter behavior either ritualistic or pastiming.

Berne's list of time structuring, remember, is more of a context grouping rather than content-based. Dr. Berne, who was a practicing psychotherapist and founder of the Transactional Analysis school of therapy, helped promote the idea that more people than just doctors had the ability to help people, themselves and others, to a well being in life. His list on time is worth deeper examination.

HOW WE STRUCTURE TIME

Berne developed this list over the course of 25 years of his therapeutical practice, both with patients and training others to be counselors and therapists. The idea that both groups behaved similarly in regard to wasting time does not go unnoticed. Few schools teach the principles of planning and execution. The closest we get to time conformity is the class bell and then what follows does not often fulfill a desire to be time conscious.

Berne distinguishes good time from bad time by observable acts of both patient and therapist. Example: Sleep is a necessary commodity in all of our lives. Most people require eight hours a night, more or less. We've all done with less during critical times in our lives, say when a loved one is ill or when waiting for a teenager to return home from a night "out."

A few individuals, because of metabolic make-up and other biological influences, have gone years on as few as three or four hours a night. Most of us know more of the other side of the coin where sleepers with 10, 11, or more hours is the norm. These "sleepy heads" are getting into what Dr. Berne calls withdrawal.

Withdrawal is an essential part of living. When the stress is too severe or the risk too great, what is within reason is to back away from the situation. When the other guy has all the guns and ammunition, that's not the time to stand up and fight—it's better to withdraw into orderly retreat and plan to attack another time. Long sleepers are probably playing with withdrawal—unwilling to face up to this situation or another.

Withdrawal, too, is a legitimate part of the health process. People, like Type A behavior advocates, tend to push and push until they are worn out and subject to what is commonly referred to as "burn out." When, and if, they learn the legitimacy and sensibility of withdrawal, they will less threaten their health and in fact will be promoting it. What Dr. Berne advocated was that each facet of structuring time be included in a thoughtful use of the minutes, hours, days, and years we are given.

Taking his research a step further, we see how often habit in our society becomes ritualistic, non-thinking behavior. Some rituals, like stress, are necessary to preserve tradition and respect for history. But excessive and slavish adherence to outdated policies and practices becomes ritualistic and inappropriate in a growing number of situations at work and at home.

No longer can women, for example, be kept from so-called "man's work" if they have the capability and desire to function as engineers, doctors, lawyers, judges, school principals, police officers, truck drivers, welders, and so forth. That ritualistic barrier has been broken for the good of all people.

At home, boys are learning to sew and cook—necessary living skills for bachelors and independent-minded young men—and do chores normally associated with "women's work." Girls, likewise, are learning what used to be considered as masculine kinds of behavior—without losing their femininity. The idea of androgynous behavior, attitudes and values will go a long way to rid ritualism from American lives. Young people will grow up using all of their God-given potential without fear of societal ridicule and scorn.

While a time-honored way of meeting and greeting friends is similar to ritualism, it's actually labeled pastiming. It's a way we can talk comfortably about the weather, sports, the opposite sex, and the latest jazz or rock recording without getting beneath the surface of a relationship. Superficial at best, it does call for ease of collecting some data—a cocktail party syndrome. Unfortunately, much of what passes as good-time sharing is fluff and non-productive.

Many sociological and anthropological reviews of American habits will reveal a deep-seeded display of our task-oriented instinct—we tend to keep busy, be in a hurry, and forever hassled. Activity, as Dr. Berne noted, is a genuine and dignified role we all play. However, it can get in the way of being ourselves when we overdo it. Workaholism is one extended form that grieves the American conscience.

Work, at the place of employment or leisure kind at home, sometimes turns into escapism—a combination of activity and withdrawal, a deadly duo. Burrowing into a hole so deeply that we miss the subtleties and nuances around us is the sad part of excessive activity.

A casual look at television network and cable programming gives you a good idea of how sports-minded Americans are. A more serious look and you'll see that it merely reflects the fact that we like to play games as well as watch them. For the most part, leisure and recreation are synonymous with healthy endeavor. Berne, in his book *Games People Play*, pointed out that gamesmanship can be destructive and a sick form of human interplay.

Spending time in setting up someone to fail or striking out at one's vulnerability is not worthy of positive and productive enterprise. Yet, this behavior can be seen at ever increasing frequency in American homes today. While bridge, Monopoly, tennis, golf, bowling, and other games are welcome respites to the dog-eat-dog world in which we live, excessive competitiveness too often finds its way into places where love and friendship should be.

Dr. Berne pointed out that our competitive instinct breeds spin-offs from games—rackets and stamp collecting. Each of us develops a "racket" to get an illicit amount of strokes from the system. For instance, someone who is continually confused demands and gets undue attention from others who must clarify situations and events. Some teenagers have "be naughty" rackets going to get attention from parents, who assuage their guilt by giving into childish behavior. Nearly everyone has a well-developed racket they've used since childhood and drag out on special occasions.

Stamp collecting, too, goes on all the time at work and at home. We save gold and brown stamps. When we do something well or nice and it's overlooked by someone, we give ourselves a gold stamp in reward of the slight. When we have enough books filled with gold stamps, we give ourselves a day off or we do something in direct affront to that person who's been missing our good intentions. After all, we deserve the pleasure.

Saving brown stamps is a little different. When the boss gives us a gig for something that wasn't our fault, we put a brown stamp in the book. Or when a parent shouts at a child for missing a chore that they haven't had time to do, the child licks the stamp with vigor and places it in the book. When enough books have been filled, we can go down to the redemption center and dump all over that inflictor of unjust gigs.

Whether you save gold or brown stamps, or both, it's indicative of a poor use of time. Life's too short to take up with sidetracks like psychological games, rackets, and collecting invidious stamps.

BEST USE OF TIME

The best use of time, of course, is being intimate. Within a family setting, being open, loving, and comforting is by far the most worthwhile and necessary component to preserving the unity of members and promoting healthy relationships. Dr. Berne did not mean sexual intimacy or love when he described his view of being close to another human. He meant being courteous, thoughtful, vulnerable to the point of access—allowing someone to get near emotionally and intellectually.

We don't advocate or want anyone to avoid the other ways of spending time—we ask for a review of how you are doing and possibly to get rid of some rituals and some pastiming in favor of opening up and sharing with those with whom you want to be close. You might be well advised to drop some game-playing so that you will have more quality time for your loved ones. To needle someone who you've always needled is easy, but it's also tiresome. What might be better is an arm around the shoulders, a quiet hug, and a considerate word of comfort and affection.

Changing those ways we spend time means changing behavior. Not an easy change to make. When you consider the alternatives—missed love and affection—it can be worthwhile.

We aren't running out of time; we're running outside of ourselves. Getting back in touch with our primary need for being intimate, loving, and affectionate is the goal. Parents, especially, can take the lead in this turn-around. Parents have the most to lose, if they don't. No time is like the present.

SUMMARY

Conflicts are inevitable in our lives and the skills to resolve those that can be are within our reach. Conflicts can be avoided, confronted head-on, or be dealt with in a creative fashion, whichever we select.

Getting and staying in focus is important if we are to make inroads into the drug and alcohol addiction arena. Fuzzy thinking leads to chemical thinking. Concentration in our natural rhythm makes for harmonious living and joyful sounds.

No matter what time it is, the time for better use of our resources can be coordinated to our natural instincts. When your timing is off, you're unlikely to be productive either at home or at work. You'll chug along a little out of kilter.

CHAPTER **8**

GETTING TO THE HEART OF THE MATTER

The arm hurt when he moved it a certain way, so he cradled it gently like a mother would carry a newborn. Tommy Ward feared the arm was broken and he'd catch all kinds of hell when he got home. **"So what's new,"** he thought.

It hadn't been his fault; after all they had permission from his aunt to climb the tree and pick cherries. He didn't count on cousin Jerry actually firing the BB gun and scaring him out on a limb.

The fall of eight or nine feet wasn't too far—he had jumped from taller places without mishap. It was disorienting as he slipped through the branches laden with ripe fruit. He didn't have a good perspective when he attempted to break the fall with his hands.

As he walked home to supper, his elbow hurt, but he could move his fingers and wrist. Tommy wasn't angry at his cousin—he always fooled around like that, not meaning real harm—going home bothered him. Mom would be soothing and comforting and Dad would yell. These diverse approaches coming from his parents were disconcerting to a boy of 9. He didn't have the ability to handle the pressure he felt from his relationship with them.

EXTERNAL THREAT

The corporate world, where most of us work for a living, faces enormous pressures from foreign competition, government regulations, litigation from various sources—raiders, merger-maniacs, aggrieved employees and the like—threats to revenue from shrinking and changing markets here and abroad, a transition from an understood Industrial Age to a misunderstood Computer Era, and only a glimmering hope that, someday, most of these external influences will be offset and somehow stabilized.

In the meantime, management thinks that if internal problems, which present an equally disruptive scenario as the external ones, could be stabilized this would be wonderful and would bring some relief to the work place. Because corporations tend to be reactive to both pressures, they wind up putting controls and limits on people—not unlike Tommy Ward's parents put on the youngster.

While corporations agonize about their plight and jolt about an emotional roller-coaster ride, a lot of people find themselves wanting to stretch and grow in this unsettled environment. Now seems like a good time to do it. The very forces that shock the corporate system also can trigger the personal system. Once excited, people react differently—some bury their heads in the nearest sand bucket and hope the threat will go away, others put their shoulders to the wheel, helping ride out the storm, while the crusaders accept the challenge and change...they grow.

COLLISION OF TWO WORLDS

When the chaos is at its zenith, that's when the two worlds collide, resulting in violent behavior: the corporation, which wants stability, clamps down on people and budgets, while the crusaders seize the opportunity to change systems, relationships, and themselves. Most people, though, aren't qualified—just as Tommy Ward was unskilled—and can't cope with the collision. They get bumped around and some get seriously hurt—only the crusader figures out the situation and escapes injury. Like Tommy Ward they can survive the short fall. Others stand around and gape. A few people react by simply putting bumper stickers on their vehicles.

One of these stickers is ironic: "I finally got it together, but now I can't remember where I put it." To many, it seems that the sardonic saying resembles their personal efforts for success, which always eludes them by being a notion or a step away. To some, the saying mimics the twists and turns of fate. Others read it simply as an interpretation of the troublesome truth.

While people are trying to get things in order—adapting their lifestyles—they are experiencing rapid social and economic change and more disruption than ever in their lives. And the political pendulum swings with little regard for the dogma that used to help order people's lives. The distraction of this lack of order leads to distress, which in turn leads to debilitation—people are getting sick of it.

As people are distracted from their original intentions, they become distressed, and the focus of their energies is diffused—they are thrown off their rhythm. The resulting stress causes illnesses and accidents that occur with alarming frequency, contributing to a national debilitation that has attracted the attention of corporations who are paying the medical bills, as well as that of the employees suffering the consequences.

STATUS OF ESCALATING HEALTH CARE COSTS

Another irony is that American industry prides itself on problem solving. The stress dilemma, though, seems to have the corporate strategists stumped. They are not adapting corporate lifestyles to cope with the severity of the health care problem. According to a U. S. Department of Commerce journal, Americans will spend a record $462 billion in 1987 to cover bills for doctors, hospitals, insurance premiums, and medical benefits. That's not counting the human misery of substance abuse. And no relief is in sight. Forecasters say the expense will continue to rise at the rate of between 18 and 20% a year. Four major factors are responsible for the escalation:

1. State-of-the-art medical technology is very expensive and will probably continue to be so.

2. Government, by slashing Medicaid and capping Medicare, has reduced its share of the burden.

3. Corporations are responsible for a population of older employees who are more susceptible to stress and illness than younger employees. Retirees, too, are living longer, and their care adds to the problem.

4. Employees take advantage of "free" benefits, especially dental and eye care, with little regard for cost effectiveness.

Health care costs have become the Sisyphus stone to American business—just as the problem seem to be overcome, it rolls back down the hill. What occurs is much like the federal deficit—before one phase of it is solved, another cost phases in to keep the toll mounting.

Then, too, a budding industry is growing around the health care cost epidemic. People at work learn more daily about the ill effects of stress and file charges against their employers whether the grievance is real or merely perceived. In response, trial lawyers by the thousands leap to rescue the aggrieved, even to the point of advertising on television. Employers respond by stonewalling and a classic win/lose conflict is set up for resolution in or out of court—at growing expense to both the plaintiff and the defendant.

Doctors play another role in the epidemic besides the initial one of costly services. They become defendants in more and more malpractice cases associated with a mounting litigiousness in our society. They must carry extremely high-cost insurance which forces some medical specialists to raise their fees, or work only on those cases which appear free of malpractice risk.

Juries have adopted a liberal bias in paying defendants and the courts seem to support such generosity. In some cases, the judgment is appropriate, while in others it appears excessive.

Insurance carriers add to the cost by raising their rates and the spiral sweeps upward and onward. Employer contributions for group health insurance alone in 1986 exceeded $114 billion, up 18% from the previous year. If you toss in the costs for worker's compensation, dental insurance, paid sick leave, disability insurance, and other health-related employee benefits, the total becomes record-shattering. Left unchecked, the outlook is glum for improvement in corporate lifestyle—this figure will likely double in five years. The cost has reached a point where it could bankrupt companies unable to cope with the rise.

John Repass, a senior vice-president at Safeway Stores, dolefully predicts that health care costs will in fact bankrupt businesses in tight-margin industries such as food retailing, processing, and supply. The threat is putting a lot of pressure on businesses that, according to bankruptcy statistics, are not good at handling the pressure. The American family farmer is one of the first victims of corporate cost pressures. No one knows for certain who's next, but you can get a good idea by looking around at factory closings, paneled downtown store fronts, and so forth.

The finger can be pointed in any direction and you'll likely hit someone who has contributed to the epidemic. Finger-pointing has a place in problem solving, but it doesn't alleviate the triggers which cause the human and economic plight.

In strictly economic terms, American industry now pays as much for intangible employee benefits as it makes in bottom-line profits. This is the first time the total benefits package cost has come close to overshadowing net earnings. In an era of deficits, it may just be the sign of the times, but it holds a hidden, even more serious cost—the human factor.

THE 120-YEAR-OLD MAN

In this country, men live 67 years on the average, whereas women live an average of 71 years. The consensus of gerontology experts is that, given all the information we now have on aging, the national average could easily be 120 years! So what's happening? People are literally working, drinking, smoking, and drugging themselves to death. If they don't die on the job, many suffer the accumulation of work-related distress and lead a morose existence in retirement. So not only are people cutting their life spans short, but they are also living their "golden years" in questionable quality.

People want to stay healthy. Look at

- the growing number of health spa registrations;
- the surge in home gym installations;
- the rise in weekend recreational get-away offers and uses;
- the spiraling sales of diet programs and nutrition supplements;
- the appeal of TV health and exercise shows; and
- the numbers of people jogging, running, hiking, climbing, working out and remaining active in various sports.

In general, Americans have developed a serious commitment to exercise and health. And this trend is more that a fad—it's a lifestyles revolution.

In fact, many Americans are showing interest in improving their health in more holistic ways. Many have learned to evaluate their values and behaviors and make changes accordingly—even in their work styles. For many workers, quality of life has replaced money as a motivating factor in making work/career decisions.

SURVEY OF THE NEW AGE GENERATION

This premise is supported by the surveyed members of the Entrepreneur's Alliance, a group of people who have forsaken the 9-to-5 way of working, opting for more flexible time spent at developing their careers. They ranked personal and family health as their number-one value. The Entrepreneur's Alliance "mavericks" left the corporate womb to pursue lifestyles more suited to their basic value system. They expressed their motivation in terms of five basic values:

- the desire to use their competencies to the fullest...to be technically challenged as well as being the master of how work is achieved.

- the determination to reach the highest quality of output and to be respected for quality . . . to have a high quality of healthiness and hardiness at home and work . . . A DRUG-FREE culture.

- to work with other competent people in a give-and-take atmosphere . . . to develop a team, community and family formula for satisfaction.

- to communicate openly, directly and freely so ideas are expressed and acted on . . . to listen so that problems are addressed before they become intolerable.

- to understand the economics of every situation both for short- and long-term implications . . . to be cost effective . . . to save enough for a rainy day.

This innovative group is the one that invented "corporate lifestyles."

Entrepreneurs were not alone in wanting these traits and conditions in their work place. Of the 300 leading employers in the San Francisco Bay Area, 99 responded to a lengthy survey from Golden Gate University's Institute for Productivity Improvement and noted that corporate lifestyle issues were at the core of their productivity and quality ills. Some of the companies are

IBM,
Hewlett-Packard,
Blue Cross,
Bank of America,
Wells Fargo,

BART,
General Motors,
Shell Oil,
Pacific Telephone,
California Casualty,
Transamerica Corporation,
Crown Zellerbach,
Liberty House,
United Airlines,
Kaiser Cement,
Xebec Corporation,
Standard Oil of California,
United Technologies,
Levi Strauss,
Local 1100 of Retail Clerks,
the VA Hospital at Palo Alto,
Alameda County Social Services,
and 77 other excellent and would-be-excellent participating organizations.

These companies agreed that values were not being exercised at work and/or people were not skilled enough to perform to their own levels of satisfaction. Each company is doing something about the trouble, but, like the federal deficit, the task seems to be an uphill struggle—the Sisyphus stone again. Despite all the good intentions, and despite being at the most advanced stage in our national educational process, the increases in white collar crime, alcoholism, drug abuse, and other infractions against self and employers mount to epidemic levels.

Crimes of violence, drug abuse, divorce, and unsettled family conflicts have risen to the highest rate in history, too. The deterioration of the nuclear family unit is being studied by sociologists, anthropologists, psychologists, and others in an effort to understand the implications and to discover possible avenues to follow for solutions. Ideas and examples in this book, which resulted from applied research, offer ways for work groups and families to be together in less conflictful ways—a community lifestyle.

Corporate lifestyles, a newly coined phrase, describes a need to which most American companies can relate. Companies which used to bury their heads in the sand when it came to social and community troubles now equate good personal habits with good work habits. And they understand that good health is linked to good profits. Enlightened managers now sense that one of the keys to this health and performance dilemma is appropriate involvement coupled with a balanced focus on economics and on the triggers of higher costs. The idea is to treat the cause, not the symptom. The corporation wants healthy people as much as it wants vital and energetic cash flow.

Employers have learned that a fit person is more likely to produce fit products and services. Soaring workers compensation claims, unstable safety records, absenteeism, and related health problems continue to pressure cost-containment and cost-effectiveness programs. To ensure the maximum use of all resources, the following features of the corporate lifestyle need attention:

1. **NEOTENY** . . . the ability to retain the exuberance of the "start-up" situation as the company matures. This is done through a positive internal and public image, reliance on professionalism throughout the ranks, and producing the synergy that comes from rational thinking and intuitive expression.

2. **CALCULATED RISK TAKING** . . . the introduction of new ideas, products, and methods often are enough for the organization to stretch itself and develop its muscle, knowing full well that some of the projects may fail. Paying research and development dues provides the time for innovation and creativity to grow.

3. **SUPPORT SYSTEMS** . . . the means to develop a harmonious and team atmosphere so that more of the work effort can be formatted into projects where work group members can focus on planning, action, and evaluation.

4. **MENTORS** . . . persons who can provide an informal and formal strategy for management succession. The more experienced managers can foster and encourage

new and younger talent through the mentor process. Mentors also model risk taking and discourage the Status Quo by advocating open and direct communications. The National Aeronautics and Space Administration, as broadcast by Barron's Radio Report, released a study recently, indicating that mentors were the most important part in developing creativity in an organization.

5. **TRANSITIONS** . . . the means for going from Point A to B, and beyond. This requires a plan. A need exists to develop a sensitivity and systems for those crisis moments a company endures as it matures. The better companies have strategic and contingency plans to help weather the unexpected.

6. **HEALTH CARE** . . . a program where successful organizations not only provide employee benefits to help defray normal health care expenses, but also often mandate a healthy, drug-free environment through thoughtful conflict resolution, wellness activities and stress management—treatment and recovery for those who need it, support for those struggling.

7. **PROFESSIONALISM** . . . the encouragement by successful companies to the dual career loyalties most employees have to their profession and the organization. These dual loyalties must be balanced to produce the commitment to quality and energy for peak performance.

8. **INTEGRATION** . . . the connection of time, focus, energy, and communications can be seen in how well-planned the individual and corporate calendars are; the introduction of shorter meetings through tighter agendas; the attention to details while keeping the big picture in mind and a structured forum for opinions and minority viewpoints. Integration leads to the development of one's potential—the most powerful force available to individuals, work groups, and their organizations.

By paying more attention to meeting personal needs, the corporation can meet its own needs. The key is improving personal productivity and linking it to corporate strategies—lifestyles adaptation for people and their employers. Without the connection, the rising-cost-of-doing-business epidemic will kill and maim more companies which fail to adjust. By adopting an integrative approach, a company will reach better economic conclusions. A single-dimension look at productivity, however, leads to an imbalanced conclusion and less of a bottom line. Economics, of course, is *the* major thread binding the corporate lifestyle. A major stumbling block for "buying in" is the difficulty in measuring this concept in all its ramifications.

FINDING AND MEASURING THE MISSING LINK

Productivity, long a critical measure of industrial effectiveness, has become a vague interpretation of what actually happens at work. The national shift in character from manufacturing to a service orientation contributes to this new mystery. To determine productivity figures from an input/output ratio used to be easy when "widgets" were the substantive output. The intangible product of a growing number of sectors of the American economy makes doing the same with the knowledge industry and services trickier. Until a better way is conceived for measuring complex contributions of creative staff, professional and management personnel, the productivity potential of this nation remains a hidden resource. When this occurs, we will again emerge as a serious world-class competitor.

Not even the most fervent advocates admit knowing the productivity impact of the computer. Its usefulness is regarded as awesome—yet no acceptable formula has been advanced for its users to visualize. Without a clear sense of its value, many people resist the computer, and its systems. Without clarity, people and their employers struggle to uncover its inevitable contributions to personal and corporate productivity.

FIX ONLY WHAT'S BROKEN

Medical science has concluded that stress accounts for most illness and accidents and, even though much hand-wringing and eyebrow-arching concern are evident, much of the work being done to rectify the situation is more cosmetic than curative, more reactive than preventive. Most medical and organizational experts know that disease-causing stress comes from work and home—for some, more at home, for others, more at work. Stress is the reason so many people are working so hard to become fit and stay that way. People are adapting the way they live; the corporation is dragging its feet.

The distress which people are experiencing, in the main, stems from being uncertain about what's expected of them. If they know the company strategic plan, they are distracted from carrying out their part of it because of continual interruptions, knee-jerk responses to problems, and other diversions. Some changes are necessary, but many are reactive—the result of faulty integration of strategic and tactical planning.

In most cases, the more personal tactical plan is not as well designed as the strategic plan. Or it simply is not designed at all—people in our culture do not like to plan their lives. Most of us react to pressures of the moment. While, on the other hand, the strategic plan receives much of the executive's attention. Because it covers the major economic resources of the organization, the boss lives by it. Another collision results when the plan is sent down the line, where lower level managers are asked to carry it out—whether they are skilled to do so or not.

While the strategic plan generally takes external factors into account, it often fails to do the same for internal competitive factors that distract people from the struggle for success. This competitive factor simply overwhelms many. The disparity between corporate and personal plans increases the growth of walking wounded. Without a clearly enunciated life and career plan, people tend to stagger and drift. As the result of a faulty or non-existent tactical plan, they become confused. They become tentative, tend to intimidate or be intimidated, get on sidetracks, or fall victim to false lures—reactive behaviors which compound an already-distressed work environment. They get drunk or drugged.

THE SAFETY NET

The connection of strategic planning and tactical action has broken down in many organizations. As competition becomes world-class, companies react to external pressures, especially in markets they once dominated, like steel, automobiles, machine tools, and midand low-technology. Imports from the Pacific Basin, where national subsidies and lower wages enable lower prices, and from Europe, where more modern plants and equipment mean lower prices, attract American buyers, especially with a strong dollar. The resulting trade imbalance adds to the confusion and distress. Bankers, too, get into trouble with loans to foreign governments, which experience raging inflation and a poor outlook for recovery.

American industry and government has yet to figure out how to plan for global economic realities. Our adversary culture is part of the dilemma. Very little synergy exists between the two Gullivers—Big Business and Big Government. They are usually on collision paths without deregulation and market realities.

What both can do, until they learn how to work in harmony, is focus on internal affairs to stop the hemorrhaging. More than 60% of American corporations have strategic plans, up from 40% seven years ago—mainly because of the lessons learned from the recent economic recession. But only a relatively few executives in each company fully understand the nuances and implications of each strategy. Government, too, at the federal, state and local levels, can cut the fat without cutting its muscle.

Those who understand the problem know it requires a systems approach, which involves everyone who works for a living. As every mystery and detective story writer and reader knows, the plot is simply a playing out of three elements—a motive, the means, and the opportunity. The systems approach is similar. It calls for

- a clear-cut knowledge of one's own motivating values,

- a set of prescribed skills to accomplish the tactical aspects of the plan, and

- a quick-step ability to adapt to changing issues and opportunities of the market place, whether it's in business, government or education.

With a plan, people can carry it up and down the organization informing, energizing, and fulfilling expectations. Without it, not enough people are deeply informed, distortions crop up, and things fail. Even with a plan, some managers and staff professionals in the organization, who must carry it out, are unintentionally kept in the dark, and become uncertain of why they are being asked to do certain actions. This uncertainty compounds the confusion, breeding distress. And, like the deficit, it grows ungainly and uncomfortably.

Other causes of stress at work are poor boss/subordinate relations, struggles between departments for capital and operating budgets, and, at the most personal level, a less than fully developed set of professional skills. Most people are simply not equipped, yet, to do more than cope with stress over the short term. Research, however, reveals that coping is not enough to avoid the devastation of stress in the long-term. A drink or a snort won't do it.

WHEN ARE WE GOING TO LEARN?

The cause and effect relationship is immutable. Yet studies done in the past ten years on stress and addiction, on one hand, and health care costs, on the other, have not been joined. The corporate insurance and benefits people tend to work on the technical aspects of the problem. Others try to support the human side of the equation with band-aids and genuine concern. Neither works well without the other. Without an understanding of corporate lifestyles, they continue to work in a single dimension. But they are learning.

To convince companies to change, even for their own good will not be easy. They may listen to the economic argument and still decide against sweeping changes. They'll resist change just like most of us do. And even if they can, a number of reasons exist as to what resistance will flare like a high school pep rally. One reason is that a great number of people distrust their own employers. Part of this problem is historical and part is our adversary culture.

People at work have been told to "be patient," "take us at our word," and similar hold-the-fort urgings, while nothing happens to change things. People get tired of waiting and don't believe the next plea. Their employer, whether in the form of an immediate supervisor or a phantom Corporate Culprit, suffers the consequences.

While corporations try to be humane, they were designed to produce "things." Managers are trained to produce goods and services. They don't come across as being as concerned as people would like, even with a plethora of benefits designed to stimulate and motivate. The truth is they don't manage human resources as well as they do technological, capital, and material resources. Noted management authority Peter F. Drucker, in virtually all of his books, echoes this idea by calling American Management "...a failure" in working out its people problems. The gap is as real and wide as the Grand Canyon, with dollars falling in as easily as snow does.

THE HELPFUL COMPUTER

A brief historical look at the transition between the Industrial Revolution and the Knowledge and Computer Era may provide an insight into the lack of full-scale harmony between people and the institutions that employ them.

The human potential movement of the past 30 years has focused on self development of millions of individuals, while few organizations have given much credence to the relentless effort of these people to find an easy-on, easy-off formula for social success and personal satisfaction. In fact, the search continues despite the organization. Corporate America prefers to concern itself with those arenas where it excels and can work for short-term success. Shareholders, venture capitalists, and financial analysts check on last year's earnings and this year's projection when contemplating a purchase or an endorsement. The pressure for short-term performance is immense. Chief executives come and go in a revolving-door syndrome, promoting the current state of distress. The hard focus is on material resources.

While, on the other hand, human resources are almost taken for granted. It's as if the corporation believes that people will surely take care of themselves once the benefits are provided. The evidence proves it doesn't work that way. Not enough easy contact and clear enough communication between labor and management occurs to make for consensus. The situation is similar to two professors of economics who can look at the same table of statistics and come up with different answers, depending on their point of view.

Getting agreement may take a while. What happens in the meantime is that the compensation bills mount and experts throw up their collective hands in dismay. We now know that the corporate technicians have not learned enough about human nature and very few understand the concept of synergy.

They don't believe, as Drucker has emphasized for 30 years, that people are the only resource of the organization that can grow and contribute more to long-term as well as short-term successes. part of the reason the technicians don't see this is because they are used to and comfortable with a more visible and therefore obvious connection to the bottom line—numbers. It is their language. They also rely heavily on verbal language and very little, unfortunately, on Erich Fromm's "forgotten language"—the mental imagery which can help excite people to take better care of themselves and perform to their potential.

In the past ten years, the American work ethic has centered on productivity. This is because our rate of growth has dropped to near nothing. Productivity, in a limited way of thinking and measuring, is still thought of as an input/output ratio of materials and man/woman-hours—content. What's being overlooked are the contributions of people and their systems—process. Part of the bypass is the difficulty of measuring these contributions. What is the value of an idea and how can you measure it when it may not bear fruit for five or ten years? Scoring of the human ration is not yet fully developed in the corporate ken.

Productivity and competitiveness, as it currently is measured, doesn't account for the new gains provided by computers and systems. And its effectiveness in knowledge and service industries has yet to be determined. It's a manufacturing and industrial tool whose potency is fading. What's needed is a technique to track both content and process.

A MANAGEMENT LESSON

Until these changes are made, the organization will remain one-sided and inefficient. Even with the passing of the Industrial Revolution, organizations have stayed close to the hierarchical model of management, the so-called pyramid or top down approach, practiced by the military, the church, and most other bureaucratic institutions. Only slight modifications have occurred such as

> **Management by Objectives** . . . a process of goal-setting that allows the managed and management to communicate over objective but limited criteria;

> **Matrix Management** . . . a process of temporary work groups established over the life of a project or program as in NASA's approach to getting work done;

> **Strategic Planning** . . . a process of establishing long-term corporate direction with changing tactical plans to achieve three-, four-, and sometimes ten-year objectives; and, most recently

> **Business Unit Planning** . . . a process which promotes the idea of a corporation within a corporation to take advantage of special operational or marketing expertise.

Organizations follow these on a inflexible path to fiscal success or failure.

More participative ideas have lingered awhile and faded after short and ineffectual trials. The mass production, assembly line advantages of the Industrial Revolution worked for a long time and greatly assisted in the challenges presented by World War II. But the world is changing today. The industrial policy in this country hasn't changed as much.

Only the computer has intruded on this lock-step, heads-down march. The computer has enabled organizations to better maximize capital and material resources, but the record is uneven, at best, when evaluating the impact on human resources. It, too, may be a Good News, Bad News dichotomy. Computer work is know to cause eye strain, back trouble and worse, as tension-related ills climb at alarming and insidious rates for those who spend hours locked-in at their terminals.

Computers also have been blamed, rightly or not, for the growing rate of dislocated workers in this country as the computer and its accompanying robotics technology takes over many of the assembly line jobs. The good news is that these are usually the dull, monotonous, and routine jobs in factories. Further positive news is the spawning of a new industry to build robots and their software systems, and to maintain both.

HOLDING OUT THE PROMISE

Despite its love/hate dichotomy, the computer may be the source of help to both individuals and organizations for a synergistic relationship necessary to design and develop healthy corporate lifestyles. Since biologists discovered that disparate parts of an organism could join and produce a sum greater than the individual parts, workers in other disciplines have been searching for ways to plan for synergy.

The Japanese discovered this idea centuries ago and count on it to produce goods and services today. It's a matter of using the whole brain, rather than relying on one side more than the other. In our culture, we have developed a dependence on the rational, logical, linear, verbal left hemisphere at the expense of the right hemisphere—the intuitive, emotional, spatial, and spontaneous.

As you read this, your left hemisphere is doing most of the work, scanning and processing the words, while the right brain watches.

If something written here excites you, upsets, or pleases you, the right hemisphere begins working while the left rests, having done its share. The transmission has occurred via the corpus callosum, a physical and biochemical bridge between these hemispheres. In this country, we need to learn how to trip back and forth without prejudice to achieve the harmony and balance that produces synergy and its productive and healthy outcomes. A full development of whole brain thought and action will enable a more developed corporate lifestyle as well.

Once we learn synergy as individuals, then we can transfer it to groups and eventually the entire organization—using both sides of the brain to concentrate on values, skills, and issues, unraveling our own mysteries.

Synergy has been in the domain of many successful people and companies in this country, whether they knew the definition or the word itself. Most of the self-made winners, entrepreneurs, and intrapreneurs (entrepreneurs who work for someone else) have discovered its magic. It's why they've been doing so well in the transition from the old to the new age. Many more need to learn the secret—which means adaptation of poor and imbalanced habits to healthy ones.

SHAPING THE CORPORATE LIFESTYLE

While millions have come to understand the computer and its worth, only a handful of Americans know about synergy—its potential remains hidden, awaiting discovery by people and their companies. Despite bringing some grief to the scene, the computer has brought **systems** to a point of legitimacy. The definition of a system is similar to the definition of synergy. And, if you squint your eyes a certain way, you may see the relationship between systems and synergy, and how systems approach appears to be the bridge between them.

Let me explain.

Systems and systems approach are new words made popular by the Computer Era. A system is a self-contained, instantaneously functioning, information-processing unit to produce efficiency. It differs only slightly from synergy in that it doesn't have a direct connection with the human element—a monumental distinction. You can define synergy as a self-contained, instantaneously functioning, information-processing organism to produce efficiency. Synergy, unlike a system, is mainly a human experience. That's observable and measurable.

Now take the definition of a systems approach: It connects machines, methods and human resources in a common effort. A systems approach links the science of technology with the artistry of men and women—a left and right hemisphere connection.

If a system is a rational, logical, and left-brained example of science, then synergy, when viewed in this context, can be an intuitive, emotional, right-brained example of art. A systems approach, then, would be the natural bridge, a techno-organic corpus callosum, if you will, to join both. So far, systems seem to be more in vogue than synergy and systems approaches. But that may be changing.

The Conference Board, an association of America's thousand or so largest private employers, recently reported its study of health care costs and came up with some short-term solutions, but nothing much for the long run. It noted, however, that "systems" and "systems approaches" were favored by top executives when addressing multi-billion dollar targets. These same executives admit to understanding and counting on personal synergy in their own lives. A futuristic few "feel" synergy can happen at work.

This limited number could grow, if a connection can be made between systems and synergy; then people will be more likely to enter honest, confrontive, and results-oriented dialogue with supervisors and managers at work and with spouse and children at home.

As companies become more familiar, and thus more comfortable, with systems, they'll be amenable to systems approaches. Chief executive officers, and some chief financial officers, who have an affinity for systems and systems approaches, will promote their use in solving perplexing issues of the organization. Chief executives see the Big Picture and welcome synergistic or collaborative relationships for their own companies.

Unfortunately, other executives often see only their segment or slice of the organization. They tend to "have their plates full" and are too busy to stop, step back, and gain a clearer perspective of issues and alliances that contribute to corporate health. Not being a part of the solution, they definitely contribute to the problems of health and performance.

Whether these single-dimension executives know the strategic plan or not, they don't know the values/skill/issues model—the backbone of corporate lifestyles. So they build a protectionist attitude which precludes collaboration and adds to internal competition, causing further distress. All of which contributes to the growing corporate health care cost epidemic.

CHANGING THE BUREAUCRATIC SYSTEM AND MIND

Nearly all professionals understand that balance, harmony, and rhythm are fundamental to success, yet few professionals in the business, academic, and government communities do much about it, except, maybe, on a personal level.

Some people are born with good balance, others have to work continuously at developing it. In either case, attention is required to keep it once you've got it. Because no one gets out of this world alive, it becomes a matter of life and death. The person who learns the secret of harmony will be more successful, enjoy life and its rhythm, and be more attuned to others. Such an individual has the earmarks of a crusader.

Conversely, the out-of-balance individual generally is victimized, or victimizes, causing more pain and grief than the balanced person. And, by virtue of that description, is likely to suffer more and die sooner. It's bred in bureaucracies.

The bureaucratic lethargy can be changed. By taking one step at a time, people can build a program to move toward their potential, enhance their work and home relationships, and, eventually, impact in a positive way on the work-place environment. All the pieces to the puzzle are on the table. It's a matter of moving them around to fit, like the Tangram, a Chinese puzzle which teaches how different shapes can produce a variety of acceptable forms. Figure 8.1 is a graphic description of the values/skills/issues model that can work for you and your group. The following detailed description explains how it works:

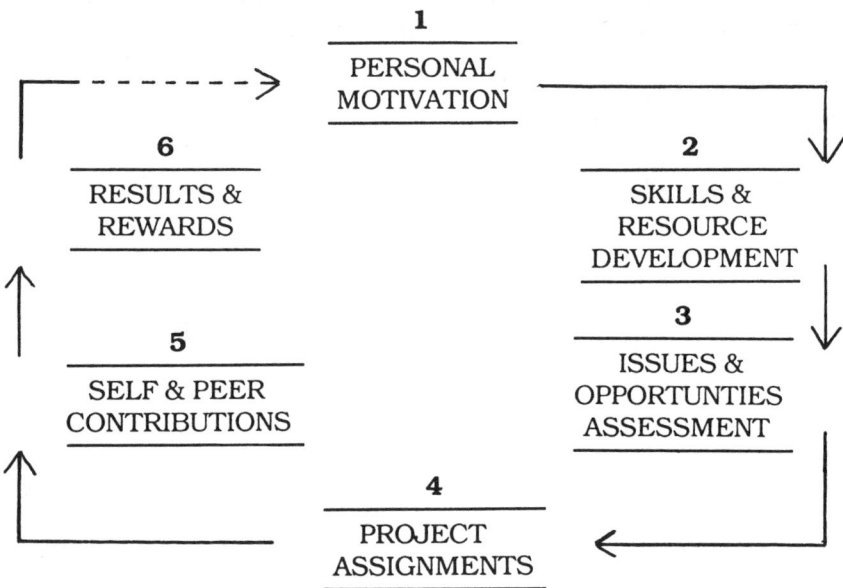

Figure 8.1. Graphic description of the values/skills/ issues corporate lifestyles model.

1. Because people are only motivated by what they value, the starting place is with a determination of personal core values. Many people are caught in guilt and fear embodiments and thus react to situations, rather than planning how to act. By understanding your own values first, and those of your peers, and then those of the organization, you are prepared for the coupling process which brings about synergy. The core values of **competence, determination, teamwork/family, communications and economics** are common to people, work groups (families), and their organizations.

2. After the values are identified and profiled, you discover the condition of the tools, i.e., skills needed to perform to new and changing expectations. Some may be good as new. Some may have been neglected, abused, or forgotten. Some will need development.

3. An assessment of the needs of people and their employers is next. It gives visibility to issues and opportunities, where you can practice your values and develop your skills. Work on this model will lead to your **potential.** You also can influence your family, co-workers, and organization to stretch and grow.

4. Once identified, these issues can be broken down to a project format which helps reduce stress within the work environment. Projects have a start, a middle, and an end, making them more manageable than ongoing, relentless work routines, which tend to become dull and boring. Projects also allow for more objective evaluation, another stress reducer. Perhaps most importantly, they lead to creativity as the interaction of people heightens such possibilities.

5. Along this path, an essential aspect is to get feedback on progress and results of what contributes to the success of the organization. Not only from those with whom you work, but from yourself, to gain credit for what you are doing. Knowing where you stand helps control stress and keeps you in focus. This process includes an evaluation index to connect health practices to professional performance—the crusaders' scorecard, which pays for performance.

6. Then, too, periodic accounting needs to occur by superiors in the organization to reward your work. Some of this will be tangible, while some of it will be psychic payment. Both are necessary for total systems performance.

7. Again the cycle repeats, providing the user with a visual framework for success. To do these things require whole brain commitment and practice, a continuous 360

degrees of calculated effort for job results and personal health.

This model is being used by many successful people and a few organizations already. Some know it by name, others do so instinctively.

SUMMARY

Distractions are leading to distress, which causes costly debilitation for people, their organizations and for society.

Individuals are being hampered by unrealized expectations, on one hand, and by dislocations on the other, which cloud the horizon for people and groups. This blocks them from productive action. People don't work well in the dark. They need some light and clarity on the features of the corporate lifestyle.

Groups such as co-workers and families are suffering from subtle conflicts and increasing violence and substance abuse on a wholesale scale with little control for solving the dilemmas. Skilled confrontation will allay the troubles.

Organizations are confronted with technological changes, shifting markets, and a transition from manufacturing to service orientation. And the burden of ever-increasing health care costs. A systems approach will provide answers to growing complexity.

For the first time on record, employee benefits costs come very close to industry's net profit. The time is ripe for reform. The reformers, who want personal as well as organizational excellence, will come from medicine, business, government, and consumer groups—joining in synergistic effort.

The corporate crusader can develop, and be developed, under a system of risk and opportunity.

The Corporate Lifestyles model is a systems approach for people who work for a living and want improved lifestyles at work and at home. Hundreds of surveyed professionals say, given the chance to learn how, they'll work at making it happen to lessen the pain and build satisfaction.

PART III
COMMITMENT...
A SYNERGISTIC PATH

CHAPTER 9

BREAKING INTO THE PERFECT CIRCLE

Studying at the Montessori school grew well on Tommy Ward. At first, he seemed reluctant. But it didn't take long for this six-year-old to adapt to the less structured environment than the one year he spent at public school. He liked his classmates and his teachers loved him—he was a breath of fresh air, exercising his natural curiosity and participating freely in every subject, even quiet time.

Tommy particularly enjoyed the well-planned field trips to the variety of interesting places that teachers took them. It was like an adventure, hunting for treasure—knowledge and answers for his inquiring and questioning mind.

One of his special friends, Bryan, stood by his side as they walked among the projects on a visit to a science museum. Tommy asked aloud, **"This waterfall reminds me of Yosemite Park, Bryan. Water's good for a lot of things, you know—watering the lawn, washing the car and, let's see, oh, yeh, my cats like it too."**

Bryan laughed and looked at Tommy, saying, **"You always have something to say about everything, Tommy. Hu, hu. You're funny."**

Later, when walking out, Tommy grabbed Bryan, made a wrinkled face and whispered in his ear, **"You're funny, too, Bryan. Hurry up or we'll have to sit with the girls,"** as they made their way back onto the bus.

IF A STAR,
THE LEAST YOU CAN DO IS SHINE

Having searched and found a new arsenal of talents and fired-up ambitions, crusaders are the kind of people who step up to be counted. They glitter with a desire to work and accomplish. Some, of course, shine brighter than others. While the bright ones seem to carry reserve tanks, some require refueling. In the case of would-be-crusaders, the fuel is a developmental plan. They need a stair step to follow and a guidance system to reach their potential.

The first step in developing your latent corporate crusadership is self-examination, following the model depicted in the last chapter. The personal search for strength and potential quickly leads to a clarification of your motives and expertise in getting things done. This chapter concentrates exclusively on how you can do this. In subsequent chapters, you continue the discovery with co-workers and senior managers and then continuing work with the family. The first step, though, is to prepare yourself quietly, thoughtfully and with a sense of expectancy—the format for synergy.

Once preparation for change begins, the individual stands alone and must risk stepping across the line into new and often uncharted territory. It's never as scary as it seems, yet many seem frozen in their tracks, like a rabbit in the road staring into car headlights. With a well-conceived plan, the journey can be a well-worth-it adventure . . . like the early explorers who found wealth and new places to live.

No one knows for certain what his or her potential holds, although experience shows that people instinctively believe good things happen once the exploration process begins. Most people starting the change process come face to face with a wall of energy that either propels them forward or deadens their will and keeps the Status Quo in place.

Researcher and writer Alvin Toffler of *Future Shock and The Third Wave* fame analyzed the dilemma and made several suggestions about self management which you can use:

- be an individual, know the contradictions of your own motives;

- gain knowledge to change those features of your life that need it;

- look around and determine where you fit best, and anchor in—stabilize what you can, drift with the rest; and

- be versatile, be adaptable, but be yourself first.

Toffler was calling for something "new," a departure from traditional answers that won't keep pace with the speed of today's society. He wasn't advocating the tearing down of all institutions, although some could qualify for demolition or serious treatment.

He was saying that to survive the individual has to take charge and not be intimidated by mediocrity and mendacity. He was calling for an adaptation, similar to the one Tommy Ward made from structured public school to the freedom of expression made possible in the Montessori setting. This is essential if corporate lifestyles is to become central to your living system. It amounts to redirecting your intensity and energy so that your strengths work for you rather than being obstacles in your path. You start by taking the self-assessment Synergy Skills Survey provided in the next section of this chapter so as to learn more about your intensity and skills.

SYNERGY SKILLS SURVEY

The Synergy Skills Survey details how your energy is working for or against you. The completed survey makes the process of lifestyle adaptation more visible and relatively easy to manage. Without this visualization, the change effort will be dinted and not as effective as possible. It's important to do the survey in terms of how you see yourself now, not how you'd like to be. That comes later. Take time now to complete the Synergy Skills Survey (Figure 9.1). After completion, score and then record your score. Interpretations are provided later in this chapter.

Instructions

Respond to the items on the Synergy Survey by marking each with a 2, 1, or 0:

A. If the item is very much like you, use 2.
B. If the item is like you some of the time, use 1.
C. If the item is unlike you, use 0.

Work through the Survey as quickly as you can without attempting to analyze or *psyche-out* the statements. Be sure to answer all of the statements and to be candid and honest.

Instructions for scoring and graphing will follow

1	2	3	4	5	6
___has solid expectations	___cynical	___slightly resentful	___can't be intimidated	___oblique/indirect	
___stubborn	___sense of tomorrow	___changes slowly	___self promoting	___is strong technically	
___investigative	___has clear direction	___political	___confident	___reflective	
___mature	___traditionalist	___calm	___suspicious	___results minded	
___can see trouble coming	___enjoys work	___seen as unfriendly	___satisfied	___favors action over words	
___practical	___occasionally cuts corners	___deliberate	___follows exact action steps	___neighborly	
___busy	___eager beaver	___linear thinker	___shrewd	___creates conflicts	
___predictable	___discontented	___indifferent	___on time	___successful	
___weighs pro and con	___puts off decisions	___turns negative into positive	___insightful	___achieving	
___domineering	___rational	___argumentative	___daring	___wary, skeptical and cunning	
___rigorous	___aggressive	___searching	___forceful	___inquisitive	
___self assured	___self critical	___realistic	___confrontive	___pioneering	
___ambitious	___thinks ahead	___likes to be tested	___wants tough assignments	___sometimes can be ruthless	
___quality	___thinks on his/her feet	___relentless	___tactless	___goal setter	
___knows limits	___obstinate	___shares blame	___follows orders	___sky's the limit	
___uses others	___aims high	___arbitrary	___keeps track	___challenger	
___delegates easily	___navigator	___comfortable with others	___can light up a room	___orderly/organized	
___sarcastic	___rebellious	___controlling	___visual	___reads between the lines	
___literal	___keeps tight reign	___bossy	___visionary	___hard/tough	
___changes mind easily	___accurate	___persistent	___defiant	___perfectionist	
___makes the pieces fit	___demands recognition	___puts things away neatly	___favors rules over ideas	___concerned with self image	
___opinionated	___inconsistent	___cautious	___thorough	___meets deadlines	
___disciplined	___agreeable	___analytical	___cagey	___patient	
___resourceful	___independent	___indecisive	___conforming	___conventional	

Figure 9.1. Synergy Skills Summary.

_accepts others _trustful _curious _stern, but fair	_work/home in conflict _demanding _self sufficient _supportive	_self confident _active listener _spontaneous _observant	_reads non-verbal behavior _research-minded _intuitive _powerful	_enjoys all competition _impressive _optimistic _quick to judge	7
_favors people over things _impulsive _poised _adaptable	_can sell anything _team builder _convincing _charismatic	_selective _likes people _I'm okay, you're okay _pleasant	_curious _enthusiastic _cooperative _tactful	_gets all input before deciding _persuasive _accepting _reflective	8
_cleans up the messes _is trusted _adamant _dependable	_decisive _talkative _unwavering _playful	_vindictive _hedges bets _keeps his/her word _unfeeling	_believes in consensus _avoids conflicts _on time _moral	_can cut off small talk _gets support _accepts all others _gets close	9
_self-motivated _possessive _sure of self _good follower	_knows own values _alert _pulls share of load _self critical	_exciting to know _lenient _stable _day dreamer	_resolves inner conflicts _considerate _nonchalant _easily upset	_emotional _relaxed/confident _into feelings _in balance	10
_delegates _intimidating _tireless _encouraging	_develops others _autonomous _willful _passive	_takes time for others _gains respect _complacent _peps up others	_handles all pressure _shares glory _thoughtful _serene	_thinks and feels equally well _stands apart _conflict resolver _easy going	11
_influences others _spirited _far sighted _inquisitive	_conceptual thinker _restless _self-reliant _pace setter	_thrives on competition _antagonistic _takes chances _high energy	_carries guilt _rallies people _seeks pleasure _initiator	_rugged individualist _laughs at mistakes _gambler _goal stretcher	12

Figure 9.1. Continued .

Scoring

After completing the survey, tally in the following manner:

1. Total the scores for each of the 12 sections. Section 1 is the first horizontal portion. Section 2 is the second horizontal section and so on. Each section contains a total of 20 items for a maximum scoring of 40 points. Write each total in the box designated 1 through 12.

2. In Figure 9.2 is a sample of how you are to place your scores onto the Synergy Skills Graph, Figure 9.3.

3. Write the scores from the Synergy Skills Survey form to the Synergy Skills Graph, Figure 9.3, on the lines above the appropriate skill.

4. Plot your graph as was shown in Figure 9.2 by plotting the appropriate values and then connecting the plotted points.

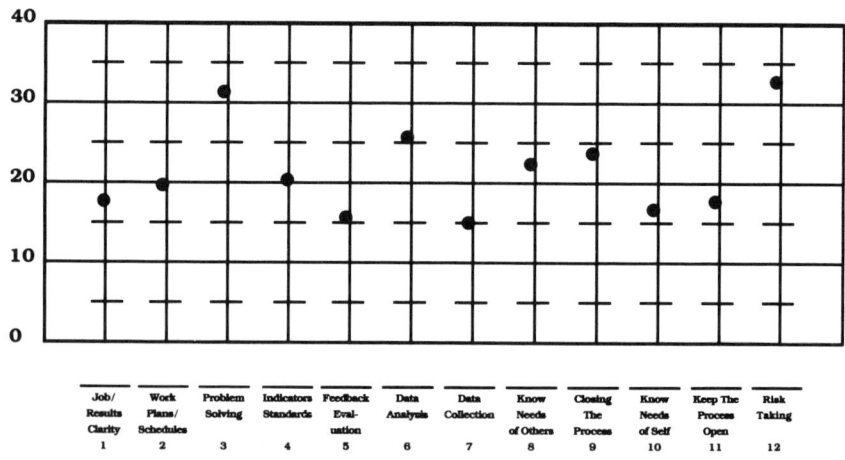

Figure 9.2. Sample of a completed Synergy Skills Graph.

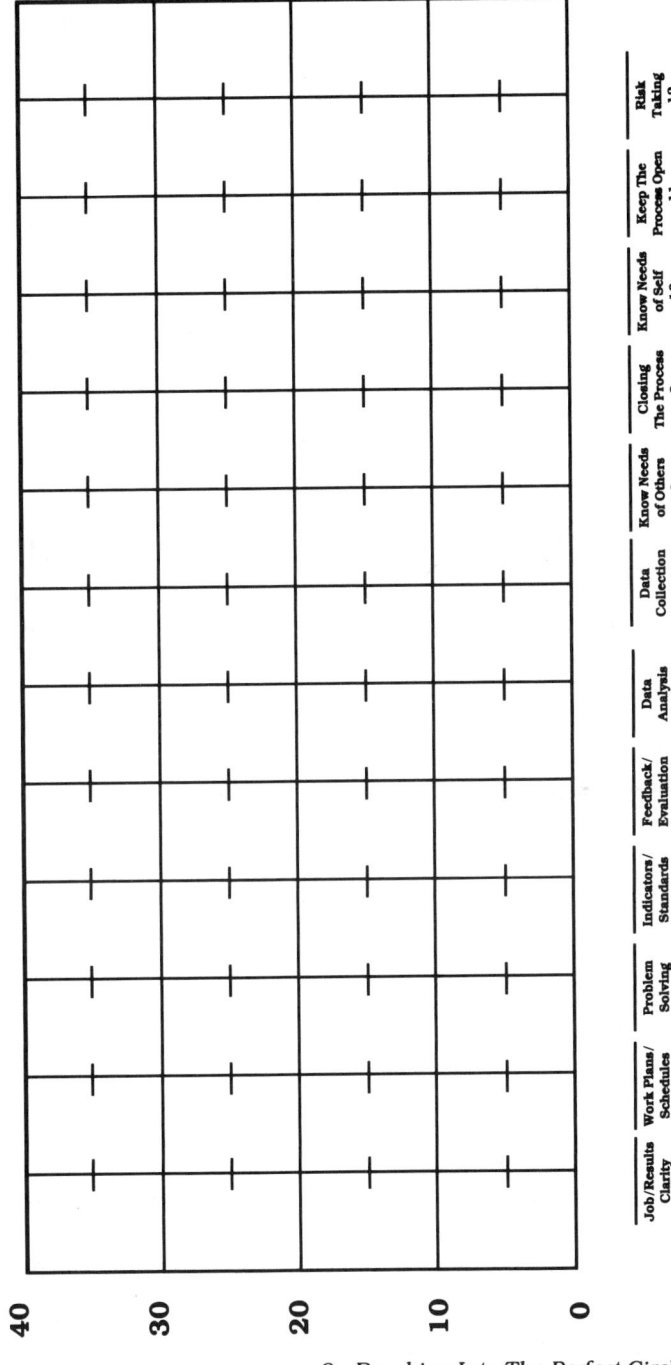

Figure 9.3. Synergy skills graph to be completed.

9 Breaking Into The Perfect Circle 213

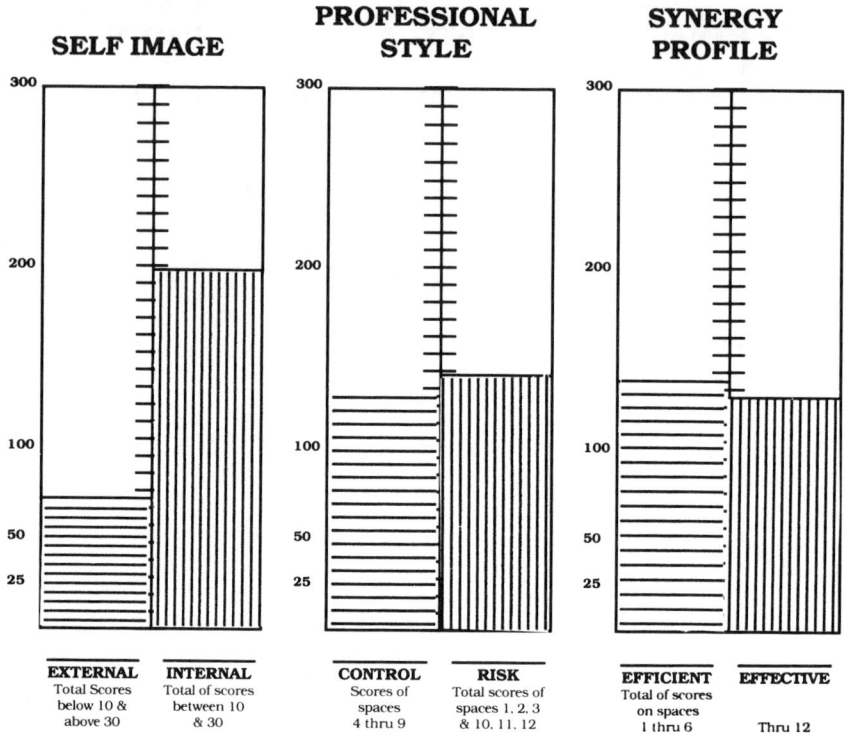

Figure 9.4. Sample of the Three Thermometer Graphs.

    5. The next step is to translate the obtained scores into a representing self image, professional style, and synergy. When finished you will have a thermometer graph as shown in Figure 9.4.

    6. Complete the **Three Thermometer Graphs** for your scores by totaling your scores for self image, professional style, and synergy and then complete Figure 9.5.

        a. ***Self Image:*** Tally those of your 12 total scores from the survey that are 10 or below and 30 and above. Enter that total on the ***External line.*** Tally the remaining scores (less than 30 and more than 10) on the Internal line.

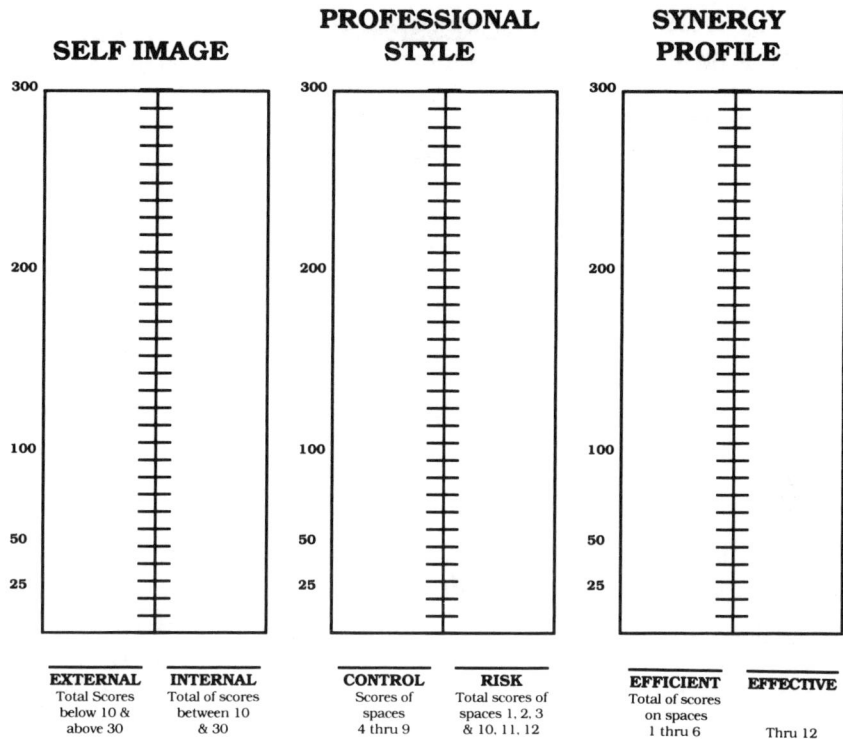

Figure 9.5. Three Thermometer Graphs.

    b. ***Professional Style:*** Tally the scores from Sections 4 through 9 and enter that total on the **Control line.** Then tally the remaining scores (1, 2, 3, 10, 11, and 12). Enter the total on the Risk line.

    c. ***Synergy Profile:*** Tally scores for Sections 1 through 6 and enter the total on the Efficiency line. Tally the remaining scores for Sections 7 through 12 and enter the total on the Effectiveness line.

7. Using different colored markers (pencils, crayons, etc.) fill the Three Thermometer Graphs, Figure 9.5, to the values indicated on the bottom lines.

Synergy Skills Scoring Interpretations

These interpretations are the result of more than 3,000 professionals taking and assessing the results of the survey. They have ranged from chief executives to engineers to lawyers to doctors to staff technicians in a wide variety of fields, both in the private and public sectors. They have agreed that peak performance comes when they have their energies flowing within the 15 to 25 levels. They also agree that stress and its resultant physical debilitations stem from operating consistently in the over-30 categories. We have given even finer definitions to the interpretations by putting them into blocks which, people tell us, have been useful in developing strategies for self-improvement.

Interpretations for Self-image

Most authorities agree that a person's self-worth is determined, in part, by the comparison of being inner and outer directed. The general belief is that **inner directed people** are more apt to understand their value system, learn from their experiences, tend to listen to themselves, and go their own way.

Outer directed people tend to go along with authority and dogma, follow the crowd, find themselves in stressful situations where it is difficult to learn, and struggle to reach stability.

A **higher Internal than External score** indicates an intellectual desire to be free of constraints, a willingness to stick with a plan or project, and a knowing of what's to be done.

A **higher External than Internal score** indicates someone who listens to others, seeks stability, and generally spends too much time and energy on matters out of his or her sphere of influence.

Scores that closely match indicate someone who is being tossed and turned by events and others.

No score in one column or the other clearly indicates a definite internal or external orientation.

Interpretation for Professional Style

Professional Style is comprised of an ***emotional need for control*** (to be in charge, to have structure and predictability) and ***risk*** (to go with the flow, to trial and error, to learn from experimenting). The control/risk configuration is based on what happens when you are emotionally committed to the situation. While the ***self-image*** configuration of internal/external scores is mostly an intellectual assessment, professional style includes one's emotional investment as well.

A ***higher control score*** indicates someone who takes charge of career and life opportunities, follows self-direction, and relies on a patterned approach to achieve. Control personalities seek comfort over uncertainty.

A ***higher risk score*** indicates someone who searches for new ways to do things; will take a flyer to solve a particularly difficult dilemma in life, work, and career; and is apt to be more spontaneous than others.

While a few points difference means much in this configuration, ***matching scores*** (two or less points difference) indicate someone who adapts well to crisis and change, can calm a disrupted work environment quickly, and is equally facile working in controlled situations and chaotic ones.

Interpretation for Synergy Profile

While the self-image is an intellectual view for yourself and the professional style is an emotional glimpse, the synergy profile is a combination of both plus some cultural dimensions. This is significant because it measures how efficient you are with things and how effective you are with people. The idea is that if you manage both well, you are in a harmonious, resourceful, and imaginative frame of mind and body—synergy.

In understanding this relationship of things and people, the general agreement is that Americans tend to score lower on the

efficiency scale, but that actually means this score is disciplined and acceptable. Since most of us will score higher on the ***effectiveness scale,*** this means we are not as disciplined there. This imbalance leads to lack of synergy. The ideal synergy score is matched on the efficiency and effectiveness scales.

An ***adequate efficiency score,*** then, generally means more comfort, skill, and interest in things. It correlates closely to ***left brain*** dominance where rational, linear, logical, scientific, and objective thinking reigns.

A ***higher effectiveness score*** generally indicates a preference for spontaneity, visual, non-verbal, subjective, and expressive aspects of approaching work and problems. It corresponds to the ***right brain.*** Because schools and work places don't encourage right brain action, these skills aren't as developed and it takes longer to utilize them well. And time is money.

Some groups, like doctors and engineers, may actually have a higher efficiency than effectiveness score because they tend to see people as things or units. Other professional groups, like teachers and nurses, generally have much higher than average effectiveness scores because they are working against such high odds for balance.

A statistical few will have close to matching scores. These are people who are well versed in using resources and dealing with others. This ambidextrous ability with skills is what brings about creativity and unexpected productivity. Let's look at the skills definition before examining the synergy graph.

Interpretations for Efficiency Skills
(Related to the need of clarity)

1. JOB/RESULTS CLARITY
(Related to the need of clarity)

The ability of knowing what's expected of you by the many people keeping track. It concerns itself with getting acceptance before starting projects as well as listening to what they want you to achieve.

15 through 25: You have a solid grasp of your job, know what is expected, and know how to measure outcomes. You keep the key people informed and gain their acceptance before acting. You can readily and easily explain your job and expectations to anyone who needs to know. This clarity sets your course and gives direction needed to insure success in the venture.

26 through 30: Same as above except that you spend a little too much time and effort at keeping others informed, or perhaps you extend the circle too wide, including those that are not directly involved in workaday projects. Be selective. Don't spread yourself too thin with alliances and allegiances.

Over 30: You are tending to be everything to everyone. This zealous approach for clarity can actually distort and cloud. Simplify your communications. Be more direct. Tell them your intentions and then get on with it.

14 through 10: Put a little more structure around your ideas and plans. Substantiate the elements of the plan. Question yourself first, then question others before you seek approval. Be more resourceful in your research.

Less than 10: You may be in a new assignment/project that calls for more rigor on your part in determining expectations. Or you may be in an old assignment that suddenly has become more complicated. In either case, find out from the scorekeepers (your boss and others) what is possible and realistic. Then add your expectations to the pile. Talk with others in similar situations or those who held your post before you. Brush up on performance planning techniques.

2. WORK PLANS/SCHEDULES
(Related to the need of achievement)

Once you have acceptance, then you can map out a time line of activities, schedules, and details of your performance. It also includes a comprehensive step-by-step resource allocation.

15 through 25: Once clear on what's to be done, you organize the pieces of the puzzle into a step-by-step action plan.

You work with budgets and deadlines, lining up the resources to fulfill the plan. Few surprises.

26 through 30: You tend to want too many answers before embarking on the work at hand. You may be scheduling too tightly and not allowing space for the inevitable. Pull back on the reins a little.

Over 30: You have a tendency to be rigid in your way of doing things. Allow for more flexibility and involve others in the planning process. By doing so much yourself you put too much pressure on the process. Make a realistic time table and share it with those who can contribute to the success of the effort.

10 through 14: You resist writing out the plan for fear it will be etched in stone and unchangeable. Not so. Write it down so others can see it. Emulate the other successful planners who visualize their intentions.

Less than 10: You rebel against structure or have yet to learn how to develop a systematic work schedule. Talk with others in the organization who have experience and success in detailing the steps necessary to get things done.

3. PROBLEM SOLVING
(Related to the need of industry)

When the plan is set, problems invariably occur. This measures your ability to quickly confront and resolve the glitches which may be technical or of a more personal nature. It can also cover inner conflicts which crop up.

15 through 25: You have reliable technical as well as people problem solving skills. You confront the zigs and zags in the plan as they happen using a combined scientific and intuitive style. You see problems as opportunities and welcome the chance to change things so everyone wins.

26 through 30: In your zeal to solve problems, you tend to over-reach your sphere of influence. Exercise patience. Wait to be asked to resolve sticky situations. Help others learn your expertise—let your experience work for you.

Over 30: Your high intensity propels you to the middle of things. Relax, count to ten, and then do it again. Learn to negotiate—otherwise you will intimidate others to a point of disruption.

10 through 14: You tend to rely too much on the plan and don't react to the snarls that crop up. Don't be tentative. Be more assertive in dealing with people and with the technical wiggles and wobbles of the system.

Less than 10: You are avoiding issues on both efficiency and effectiveness levels. Get some help to learn systematic approaches to analyze and predict outcomes. Be forceful in asking for assistance in this critical area of your development.

4. INDICATORS/STANDARDS
(Related to the need of integrity)

Whatever the work effort, certain keys keep the project or program in the groove. After debugging a system, that's the time to implement how the prototype can be fulfilled over the longer term. These measures should be realistic and not artificial or arbitrary.

15 through 25: You have strong abilities in breaking work into bitesize chunks (indicators) and setting quality goals (standards) for the finished product or service. You are realistic, not expecting the impossible. You control resources well because of this stability.

26 through 30: You get momentum going but run too hard and fast for those around you. They tend to be off balance because of your intensity. Develop a quality index that fits the situation and keep others on a firm footing with you. Ease up a bit.

Over 30: You are running the train into roadblocks by expecting too much of yourself and those around you. Take off the engineer's hat and let someone else blow the whistle and ring the bell. Give others a chance to get aboard and ride to the end of the line. They'll show their capabilities along the way.

10 through 14: You need to examine the system and see where the pieces fit. Then you can demand more from the people involved in getting work done. Once you see work as a block diagram, you will better understand spatial relationships and how they help achieve results.

Less than 10: You have become too dependent on others to set the pace. Be more forceful in organizing work so it hits the quality target. Concentrate on blocks of work instead of the nitty gritty details. Find someone who knows the systems approach for optimum use of resources at your disposal.

5. FEEDBACK/EVALUATION
(Related to the need of control)

In tracking work flow, the need is for ongoing communication in a positive and unbiased way with those doing the work. When it's visual, it has a double impact in keeping the flow smooth. Periodic evaluation helps reward peak performance behaviors.

15 through 25: You talk straight, are fair in scorekeeping, and show appreciation for a job well done. You keep communications open on how things are progressing and are supportive of those who request help in reaching goals.

26 through 30: Because of your intensity, you tend to be inconsistent with feedback—some you lavish with praise, others see the stingy part of you. Feedback is a two-way communication; let others in so all know what's being measured.

Over 30: You stop people in their tracks with your feedback and intimidate them. On the other side of it, you extend the process too far by requiring an overabundance of feedback on how you're doing. You could be more helpful by being more specific in your dialogue on how to keep the train on the track.

10 through 14: Be more emphatic about the progress of projects so people know where they stand. Don't be reluctant to share what you think and feel. Be more visual in your communications. Ask for updates.

Less than 10: A system for priorities would aid you in getting satisfaction out of work. People want to be appreciated for what they do, you included. Make your needs known so others can assist you in being more explicit in measurement and feedback.

6. DATA ANALYSIS
(Related to the need of curiosity)

This is the ability to sort out the intelligence, data, and other information in an unbiased, research-like mode to determine what went right and wrong. It could include post mortems, critiques, and thoughtful review of plans.

15 through 25: You assess data, information, and intelligence from a variety of sources well. You read between the lines and the writing on the wall. You have a sense of here and now along with a penchant for the future. You are good at uncovering best options for diverse situations.

26 through 30: While you generally come up with solid solutions, you also tend to over-analyze. This perfectionism extends the process, consuming time which causes delays and frustration. Find reasonable sounding boards for your assumptions.

Over 30: Your desire to dot all the I's and cross all the T's wears thin after a while. Being right isn't always best for the group. Allow others to input while the data are being massaged. Be more spontaneous and work more quickly.

10 through 14: You come up with some right answers but some question your methods. Tell them about your scientific inquiry. Settle their doubts to convince the skeptics.

Less than 10: Develop a systems approach to analyzing data. Become a detective about information. Look around for clues. Critique meetings and events to practice this skill. Talk to those who seem good at it. Curiosity may have killed the cat, but it will help you perform better.

**Interpretations for Effectiveness Skills
(See Figures 9.3 and 9.5)**

**7. DATA COLLECTION
(Related to the need of trust)**

Much of the data needed to perform to high standards and to reach one's potential are stored with people, not in computers or files. This score measures your ability to access data in a technical and personal fashion including the clues and nuances that make up normal people to people relationships.

15 through 25: You exhibit a determination to gather information on both sides of the issue or question. By being relentless in inquiry, you have learned who to trust and who not to. You uncover data from the technical banks as well as from people.

26 through 30: While a vigorous data collector, your enthusiasm often disturbs others who may want to settle for less. Relax the drive but don't relax the objective. Spend more time in creating trust with those involved in the process.

Over 30: Your fervor for getting all data is too much for most people, especially if little trust has been established in the relationship. Give yourself time limits in which to build a data base. Be more creative in seeking information—pressing isn't the only way to access data.

10 through 14: You usually get the data, but could be more skillful in doing so. Be more assertive; don't take no for a final answer even if it creates conflicts. Conflicts can be positive if you work at relationships. Patience is a virtue but sometimes it can be seen as apathy.

Less than 10: Learn to access the system by developing investigative techniques, especially around people. Skepticism can be healthy but not if it immobilizes your efforts. Learn to research. Model yourself after dynamic, forceful, and effective people in your company.

8. KNOW NEEDS OF OTHERS
(Related to the need of intimacy)

Fundamental to your success is determining what others want from their time and effort spent at work. It also measures your skill at developing team or group direction based on their skills, ambitions, and commitment.

15 through 25: You get to know people easily, can work at group consensus and gain support for difficult projects. You can bond people's needs with the needs of the organization. This sense of community helps shape productivity and quality of work life.

26 through 30: You go out of your way to find out what others want but tend to become too involved in their routines. Concentrate more on the stated goals and objectives or help others uncover them. Spend less time on rituals. Don't worry about hurting feelings—take care of business.

Over 30: You are involved too deeply with too many people. It takes a toll in time, energy, and communications. Limit yourself and your involvement. Don't get caught in global issues—stick to the work plan.

10 through 14: Most of the time you know the people and their needs and you can work toward consensus. When you fall short, it's because of lethargy. You don't want to get too close and tend to overreact. Test yourself by putting more of yourself into the process.

Less than 10: You tend to be self absorbed and miss out on learning from others. Relying on self is good but when it causes you to miss out on synergistic opportunities, you lose. Develop a support group, trust its members and gradually build comfort with being close to others.

9. CLOSE THE PROCESS
(Related to the need of generativity)

This ability allows you to put an end to a wandering discussion, make a sound decision, and not lose sight of the organizational objectives as well as more personal ones. It means being able to get close to others without losing yourself in the arrangement.

15 through 25: You listen, search out, and probe even the passive people to make decisions in a timely and concise manner. You are adept at wrapping up projects, meetings, and encounters. You get close to people to figure out how to create long term alliances which builds a foundation for the future. This assures that the place will be left better than when you got there.

26 through 30: You get closure most of the time, yet overly protect some people, and are harsh with others. This inconsistency delays decisions, or they are made at someone's expense. Be more visual in expressing yourself. Check perceptions with others.

Over 30: Don't spend so much effort on the process. Cut off dialogue when it's time. Plan fewer and shorter meetings. Try the 30-minute meeting formula. Develop more visual formats for decision-making, such as chalkboards and flipcharts.

10 through 14: You tend to have the answer in hand while asking for input. This foregone conclusion pattern turns off people and deflects satisfaction. Be patient enough to let the process work and react less to control needs. Let others struggle with coming up with best solutions.

Less than 10: You tend to be a loner and enjoy working alone. This isolates you from new ideas and creative energy. Exert your effort on gaining consensus and work from a timetable. Take a chance on being heard.

10. KNOWING SELF NEEDS
(Related to the need of self identity)

This measures your insight and understanding of your own drives, aspirations, and motivations. It also scores you on how well you "get up" for performance when you may not be inspired.

15 through 25: You identify with your work. You know who you are, where you are going, and how to get there. In spite of sudden shifts and turns, you keep in focus and know the direction to take. The personal balance you exhibit stabilizes others.

26 through 30: Although you know yourself, you tend to want to know more. Rely more on your own good judgment in different situations. Be adaptable but don't shape yourself to someone else's expectations. Take each opportunity as it comes and play the role you identify with.

Over 30: You can't be all things to all people. Believe in your talent. Don't spend time second-guessing yourself. It's better to test what's at hand. No one responds to a chameleon; the changes are too abrupt. Be yourself and less of a superman or superwoman.

10 through 14: You have a few doubts about yourself, but who doesn't. Stay with the comfortable roles. Try experimenting a little more, though, and you'll find that you don't have to change all that much to be successful. Even major leaguers adjust their stance from time to time.

Less than 10: Being asked to take on new assignments and tasks can be confusing—but try a few. Ask for help from more experienced people around you. Take on new challenges, one at a time. Give yourself time to grow. You will flourish once you do.

11. KEEP PROCESS OPEN
(Related to the need of autonomy)

When you have all the prior skills down cold, you still need patience to allow others to generate input on what's happening or planned. This often takes too much time and how well you do it within limits tells the measure of success.

15 through 25: Being your own person, you allow others to be like-wise. This facilitates harmony at work and enables you to withstand the pressure to act before the time is right. Without the hurry-up attitude, you create a space for skeptics to overcome their doubts and help you turn negatives into positives.

26 through 30: You want everyone to be heard but you have a tendency to prolong the process. To listen and observe at the same time is difficult, but practice it. Help others resolve their conflicts by resolving those that confront you.

Over 30: Be more dogmatic about time limits and about people coming prepared to meetings. Collaboration is great but so is doing one's homework. Be more selective about whom to rely on and make it a point to reward those who work within established limits. Don't rush the relationships but speed up the activities.

10 through 14: You work well with groups but often go with first conclusions. Be more patient, especially at drawing out those who tend to keep away from controversy. Learn to negotiate without stifling conflicts. Much that is hidden generally turns up in the heat of a face-off. Be prepared for emotional outbursts which can lead to creative solutions.

Less than 10: You stick with conventional views about work. Times are changing and you can change with them by showing a concern for people and their views. Confront others to learn more about success at work. Be more assertive and willing to deal with emotions. In the long run, you and they both win.

12. RISK TAKING
(Related to the Need of initiative)

This measures your ability to put stretch in your life and work goals, to discover your potential, and to innovate around the issues at work. It cycles back to the No. 1 skill, which is how well you understand expectations. It measures how well you expand current limits, raise standards, reduce costs, and improve methods while keeping the current structure in place.

15 through 25: You have a healthy appetite to be different, to try new things, to innovate, and to be creative. You have vitality, strong will, and can explore uncharted paths with verve and excitement. You look for ways to cut costs and create cohesion at work. You're on your way to your potential.

26 through 30: While you thrive on taking chances, you may push boundaries too soon while you test yourself. This takes a lot out of you because the system tends to be lethargic. It causes others to wonder why you're in such a big hurry. Get some allies to test out the waters with you.

Over 30: You are a gambler and competitor. You look for open windows to jump out of. Check on the safety net before you leap. You lose sight of the dangers in your rush for enterprise and success. Burnout is a step away if this pattern becomes habitual.

10 through 14: You try new things once in a while, but you don't really like to make waves. Being cautious has its place but so does research and development—experimentation. Pioneer a new plan or back someone who has one. Play with ideas and suggestions before setting them aside. Accept change willingly.

Less than 10: As a traditionalist, you prefer to play it close to the vest. Someone has to ante up to build the pot. Read up on venture management and talk to strangers, make new friends. Don't stay in the shadows. Work on building your confidence by helping support others who are more forceful.

THE ROAD TO PEAK PERFORMANCE

In Figure 9.6 is a graphic description of potential indications according to the intensity (score) received on each of the twelve Synergy Skills Survey.

The first thing to look at is the intensity of the total graph by reviewing your Synergy Skills Graph, Figure 9.3. Are all the scores above the 20 line? All over 30? Only the right brain scores over 30? Some under 20, some over?

> **All scores over 30**—The conclusion is that you must figure out ways to relax as soon as possible. This scoring indicates excessive stress and strain on you and those in your environment. These scores above 30 call for a meaningful plan to redirect time and energies so you can recharge more often.

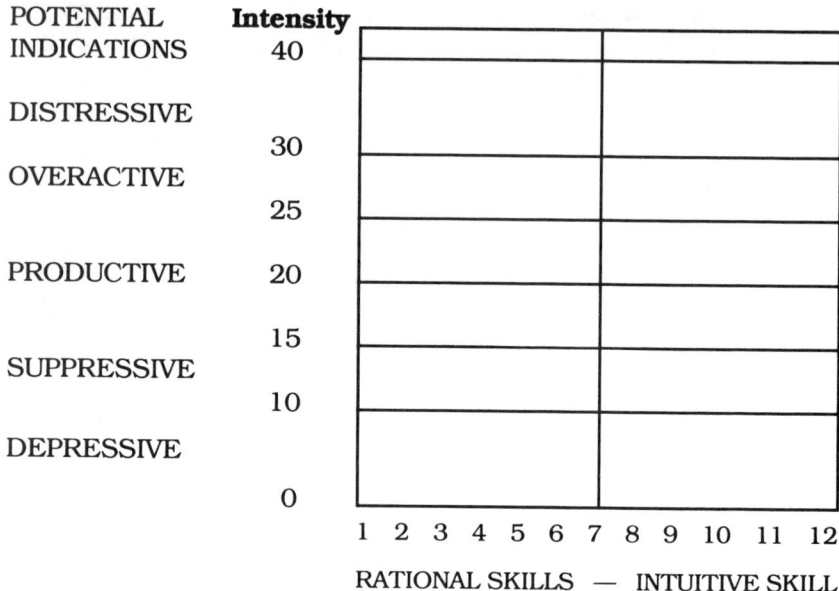

Figure 9.6. Synergy profile—a schematic representation of potential indicators as shown by intensity in each of twelve synergy skills.

All scores under 15—You can start by examining why you aren't more committed to the organization.

20 ± 5 Scores—If you have scores that dip and weave up and down the 20 line, you've developed good use of your energies and are getting as much back as you're investing.

Scores of 26 through 30—Scores mainly in the 26 through 30 range are a little too intense, and can benefit from planning to relax more than you currently do.

Scores of 10 through 14—Scores in the 10-14 range indicate a call for more involvement and perhaps more time spent communicating and relating with those who count.

Scores Less Than 10—These call for a serious upgrade of your current approach to work.

Range of Scores—One's score may range from one number one day to a different number another day. That range is reflective on one's zone. Also if the score is approximately the same from day to day. Then one can identify the potential indications (Figure 9.6) from that range in intensity scores or intensity zone.

Distressive and Depressive Zones. Scores of 30 to 40 and 0 to 10, respectively, are indicative of too little and too much energy displacement. Like a traffic light, they mean *STOP*. The distressive zone indicates an excessive use of energy that over prolonged periods concludes with burnout. The depressive zone indicates so little energy that it's tantamount to psychological depression, or burn-out. It is generally a stage that follows long periods in the distressive zone.

Overactive and Suppressive Zones. Scores of 25 to 30 and 10 to 15, respectively, illustrate a use of time and energy that is curtailed on the low end and excessive on the top side. Again, like the traffic signal, they mean *CAUTION*. The overactive zone indicates excessive energy and time spent on a specific skill, either through overkill or because situations continually arise demanding such frenetic participation. The suppressive zone generally means the individual has not fully developed specific skills (or the underlying character traits), or is holding back because of previous negative experiences.

Productive Zone. Scores of 15 to 25, is in an arena that allows for appropriate input of time and energy which produces the outcomes sought and satisfaction resulting from balanced exchange. And, of course, it means *GO*. Scores in this range indicate a development of personal abilities to meet existing conditions in a normal and healthy manner. These scores follows Julius Erving's example of playing basketball-flowing from a relaxed 15 through an alert 20 to a forceful 25 and back. It's the corporate crusader zone.

While the class of professional managers and staffers tends to operate in the Productive Zone, most do not. They work at fever pitch because many corporations reward such behavior. A close look at excellent companies indicates a growing awareness that high drive and high energy may have limitations, especially if they continue unabated for a long time and turn into habit. To avoid this frenetic trap, the synergy profile provides you with options to revamp your personal energy system so you are operating at peak energy levels for given situations.

Support for this adaptation comes from Dr. Friedman's research, the studies from Stanford Research Institute, and others who have looked at Type A behavior. The new theories talk about balance and harmony of energies. These energies can be recognized in successful people who throw themselves in, pull themselves out—allowing time for a recharge. Winners and warriors establish a positive, natural rhythm, reducing the risk of burnout.

GETTING TO KNOW YOURSELF

Now very many companies have structured work for people so they can establish an energy cycle that has positive ups and downs. This is generally left to chance, a de facto dismissal of planned change. Left to chance, the energy will likely turn to stress in a pessimistic culture.

Then, too, some people attempt to avoid stress at all costs, and practice avoidance behavior. They block out most emotional triggers and rely mainly on rationalizations to live their lives. These people populate industrial, commercial, and governmental bureaucracies.

Avoiders play safe, keep low profiles, and back away from any situation or person which might develop into conflict. They play a game of passive/aggressive behavior, switching from no interest in a subject to heated emotions without taking any positive action to change the situation. You can visualize their swings on the Synergy Profile chart going from 10 to 30 and back again. While they think they are successful in avoiding stress, they also avoid the satisfaction that comes with productive living. And the reality is that they don't avoid stress after all. Passive/aggressive behavior promotes distress at several levels.

That's why it's important to know your tendencies, so you can maintain what's working productively for you and adapt the rest.

What's also important is knowing your intensity levels, Figure 9.6, because medical scientists tell us stress is cumulative, and unless you do something to get rid of it, stress clings to you, physically. It generally returns to a familiar place, and that's a weak or damaged spot on your back, neck, shoulders, legs, stomach, arms, head, or wherever it can gain a foothold and cause trouble. It may appear as tight or pulled muscles in the neck and shoulders area, lower back pain as it breaks down musculature, or as nervousness, headaches, and irritability.

Without regular release, the stress keeps snipping away at good health. Stress eventually becomes a body armor, trapping good health inside.

After determining your current status, the next step to good health and productive performance is to make a commitment to be more involved in working through the inevitable dilemmas at home and work. When you look around and see successful people, they get involved in personal and emotional matters all the time, often with the style and grace of a world crusader—a 15-to-25 rhythm, Figure 9.6—not with passive/aggressive swings from a low 10 to a frenetic 30-plus.

VALUES SURVEY AND PROFILE

With enough knowledge, educators used to think, people will change from bad to good habits. The efficacy of that assumption has long been shown to be a product of defective thinking. People need more than knowledge to change habitual behavior. They need a system which includes:

- basic motivators,
- support for the proposed change,
- time to practice the new behavior,
- feedback on the new behavior, and
- a reward for doing the change.

That is why the **Values Profile** is the next step in the system.

While the ***Synergy Profile gives you a conceptual look at your behavior in terms of skills, the Values Profile provides for you directions to understand your motivation and options for use.*** It spells out in clear terms where you are being satisfied or dissatisfied with your core values of competence, determination, teamwork, communications and economics. Upon completion of the **Values Survey** in Figure 9.7

you will be a step closer to linking your motives to your skills so you can create the lifestyle you want in order to reap the benefits of your potential.

The Values Survey in Figure 9.7 is not intended to be a scientific study of your belief system, but it can provide an easy and non-threatening way to assess how things look to you today. People in a hurry often forget to stop every once in a while and check their own equipment. As Arnold Palmer said in the Pennzoil commercials, "It's good to check the old equipment frequently." The surveys are a straight forward dialogue with someone you may have overlooked as a valuable resource . . . you. If you prefer to do the written work after you've finished this chapter, so be it. Your reward will be a personal experience similar to the give-and-take rhythm that successful crusaders model.

Statement	WORK	HOME
Instructions: This values survey will help assess your perceptions of values at work and home. For each statement as frankly and openly as you can, record a scale number for work and another scale number for home. Use this scale: Always, 5; Usually, 4; One-half the time, 3; Infrequently, 2; Never, 1.		
1. We have well-defined objectives, audits and time lines for what we plan to do.	_____	_____
2. People regulate their workload rather than having too much or too little to do.	_____	_____
3. I maintain a smooth routine despite changing or new priorities.	_____	_____
4. I react well to crisis and develop fire-fighting systems for crises.	_____	_____
5. We get things done despite serious and severe complications.	_____	_____
6. People know their motives and are self-directed.	_____	_____

Figure 9.7. Values survey instrument.

Statement	WORK	HOME
7. I am clear about what's expected of me.	_____	_____
8. I'm enthusiastic, in shape, and not "burned out."	_____	_____
9. We confront each other to resolve conflicts.	_____	_____
10. We reward teamwork as well as we reward individual contributions and effort.	_____	_____
11. I'm supported for my ideas, plans, and actions.	_____	_____
12. I support others even if I doubt the outcome.	_____	_____
13. We communicate rules/practices/policies in a timely and useful manner.	_____	_____
14. We talk openly about all problems.	_____	_____
15. I know how others see me on all issues.	_____	_____
16. I accept constructive criticism graciously.	_____	_____
17. We spend resources wisely, getting full value.	_____	_____
18. We have solid understanding of economics.	_____	_____
19. I'm expected to control budgets and costs.	_____	_____
20. I spend and save with equal facility.	_____	_____

Figure 9.7. Continued.

Scoring

After scoring and interpreting you will be able to understand your perceptions of your organization, your work associates and peers, your immediate supervisor, and yourself. You can also compare the similarities and differences at work and home. Start by tallying the scores.

	WORK	HOME
Total Score Tally the total of the 20 items.	_____	_____
Scores on Five Core Values		
Tally items 1 through 4, Competence.	_____	_____
Tally items 5 through 8, Determination.	_____	_____
Tally items 9 through 12, Teamwork.	_____	_____
Tally items 13 through 16, Communications.	_____	_____
Tally items 17 through 20, Economics.	_____	_____

Scores on Four Stages of Relationship

Add items 1, 5, 9, 13, and 17. The organization.	_____
Add items 2, 6, 10, 14, and 18. Co-workers.	_____
Add items 3, 7, 11, 15, and 19. The supervisor.	_____
Add items 4, 8, 12, 16, and 20. Yourself.	_____

Five Core Value Definitions

Researchers such as Maslow, Peters and Waterman, and others insist that values are the true motivators. Here we examine the five core values which, once understood, can lead to balance and harmony at work and home. These values are as follows:

> **Competence**—a technical ability to achieve, coupled with a sense to work well with others in a timely manner.

Determination—the willingness to strive for quality with an intensity and focus appropriate for the occasion.

Teamwork—giving and receiving support to and from co-workers, friends, and family for ideas, plans, and actions.

Communications—being timely and direct in reporting progress, problems, and results through a two-way dialogue.

Economics—having a feel for what's behind the numbers, being cost-conscious, and knowing the way to the Bottom Line.

Scoring Interpretation

These interpretations have been summarized from several thousand people who have taken the assessment and discussed the meaning in their lives. They may be as useful to you.

For Total Score

90 and above:	The organization (work environment) is in a good place, has systems in place and uses all its resources to the optimum.
80 through 89:	While generally strong and healthy, a few areas call for attention.
70 through 79:	The organization (work or home environment) tends to mediocrity and several factors require improvement.
60 through 69:	Decline has been evidenced. Things are not as they once were. Much attention and effort will correct the situation.
Under 60:	Opportunities for improvement abound. Fences need mending—a top down assessment is in order.

For Five Core Values

Competence

18 through 20: You are being fully utilized on a technical as well as on a personal level. Harmony is in nearly every facet of your work or home life.

15 through 17: You are using all your skills, in the main, but patches of underutilization cause a little frustration.

13 through 14: You'd like to see some changes. Some obstacles mar your road to progress. These obstacles could be temporary or you may have some conflicts to resolve.

12 or less: You are somewhat dispirited with how you are being used, or not being used. The frustration is such that you need to correct the situation soon.

Determination

18 through 20: You are riding the crest of success and take care to achieve goals and ambitions. Your enjoyment is obvious and the rhythm seems to be flowing well.

15 through 17: You are realistic about what's possible to get done but once in a while you may drive too hard—this tends to cause others to resist you.

13 through 14: When you get caught in the middle of a conflict, you let others influence the way things go. This behavior is causing skepticism within the group.

12 or less: You're feeling a sense of powerlessness as the events rush by you. You have

lost some of your old steam as a result of it. The time has come to recoup.

Teamwork

18 through 20: Your ideas and concerns attract the right kind of attention and support. You stand by co-workers and friends and they admire you for it.

15 through 17: You have the knack for getting others to go along with you, but once in a while you let the chips fall where they may.

13 through 14: Lately you find working with the group more difficult. Rejection of ideas seems to be the theme. Get to the bottom of it.

12 or less: New ideas seem threatening nowadays. The trend towards isolation which seems to exist must be broken if things are to get better.

Communications

18 through 20: You speak frankly, openly, and when it counts. Your comments help others know where you stand and where they stand with you. They trust what you say.

15 through 17: You are not bashful and generally say what is on your mind. Sometimes, though, your telling it like it is upsets others. Take more time in giving the rationale for your input.

13 through 14: You sometimes soften your message to avoid hurting feelings. Others see this as compromising and don't always get your meaning.

12 or less: By avoiding confrontation, you present a fuzzy picture to others. The air needs to be cleared and more direct meaning put into your words.

Economics

18 through 20:   You meet or beat budget and cost targets with pleasing regularity. This consistency pays off in both short and long term.

15 through 17:   You can keep the ship afloat in good or bad times with a keen eye for the Bottom Line. Once in a while you miss the big picture and costs creep a mite.

13 through 14:   Putting a fence around costs is not as easy for you as it might be. Cost containment is a project worth more of your attention.

12 or less: Things are getting out of hand quickly. The need for appropriate controls and a clear understanding about money matters would help solidify the scene.

For Five Stages of Relationship. When interpreting the score of how you perceive the organization, your co-workers, your supervisor and yourself, use the following scale, which corresponds to the Stages of Relationship diagram in the text. For example, if the score for co-workers is 22, it means that you have a synergistic relationship going from your point of view. If the score for your supervisor is 11, it means that you are skeptical of the relationship—a severe breach any way you look at it. The scale score and meaning are as follows.

22 through 25: A definite healthy and synergistic situation.

17 through 21: A constructive, confident work atmosphere.

13 through 16: An optimistic and generally satisfying environment.

9 through 12: A wary and skeptical aura pervades here.

Less than 9: The Status Quo reigns and not much happens.

VISITING AN ATTIC

Deborah Elkin decided she wanted to know where she was. She knew she had a lot going for her, wasn't quite sure where she wanted to go, yet something rubbed her nerves a little raw and a voice kept saying, *"It isn't right. It just isn't right."*

A widow with two teenagers, Deborah managed a posh health spa in San Francisco. While crossing the Golden Gate one morning, she felt how heavy the strain of being super mom was and believed she was about to have a heart attack. *"How could a 35-year-old health nut like me have a heart attack?"* she wondered. A few days later, after having time to reflect, she was glad the scare prompted the self examination that followed.

Deborah took the *Values Survey and Synergy Skills Survey* provided earlier in the first part of this chapter. She discovered that her lack of clarity about life and its future for her was causing undue stress. This was compounded by the grief her family experienced at the sudden and unexpected death of a husband and father. This was reflected in scores well above acceptable norms in all categories, especially those emotional skills necessary for working with people.

Putting two and two together, she first opted for a much-needed Mexican vacation, and then took the planning time needed to develop a path to follow for personal and professional direction.

As with so many people who "see" their profiles for the first time, Deborah reacted swiftly and surely after realization sunk in. Without doubt the scoring was accurate, it reflected just how things had gotten out of hand.

"I felt like huge stones had been lifted off my chest, back, and shoulders. The relief was immense. Once I knew I was doing a lot of the pressure to myself, or rather not doing enough for myself, I could breathe freely again. The sudden shock of my husband dying, the grief that literally enveloped the children and me, the cloud that settled right in our living space, all seemed overwhelming. It was so thick and so heavy. I had a lot of sorting out to do, but the self assessment helped clarify where to begin the process."

"When I looked at those scores and read what they meant, I gasped and just shook my head from side to side. I probably even clucked—tsk, tsk. . . how true it is. Without that insight from these surveys, I don't know how long, if ever, it would have taken me to get clear."

What Deborah learned, basically, was that she was giving more energy than she could possible get back. This uneven exchange can go on for a short time with no adverse side effects. If it goes on indefinitely, dire consequences follow. Like a finely engineered automobile that runs out of oil, she was operating instinctively but on a destructive path.

Her usual business acumen, which had held her in good stead through several successful ventures, was stale and flat. Dominated by the reflex action for continued achievement and success, she propelled herself into work with the usual vigor and drive, but the result was mainly motion with little forward movement. That's what gnawed at her.

Graphically, Deborah's Synergy Profile is shown in Figure 9.8; it looked like this.

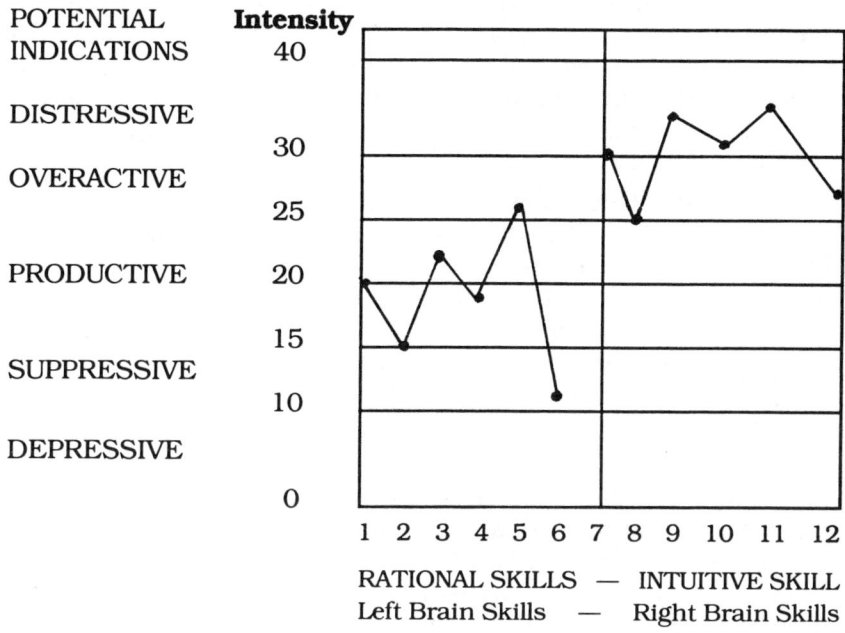

Figure 9.8. Deborah's synergy profile.

Most of us have a normal energy cycle that flows from a central point to a peak to a low back to the center, a natural rhythm that allows us to keep in balance. This cycle repeats until something or someone intervenes and causes temporary stress. At an approaching stressor, we may then shoot up to a 27 or 28. If it is really stressful, like an unexpected call from the boss about a project blow-up, it zooms into the 30s.

Again, if these are temporary and we relax into the Productive Zone, then we need not worry. However, when this cycle is repeated several times over several months, then we can expect to have problems. In the case of Type A behavior—an habitual intensity that has built up over the years, the scores stay over 30 in the Distressive Zone and with rare moments in total apathy the scores are in the Depressive Zone.

Similarly, in cases of prolonged stress, a person may experience euphoric highs changing to baleful depressions and back again. In severe cases, the highs eventually diminish, leaving the individual sapped, unable to replenish energy. The person exhibits alternating patterns of apathy and anger, loss of concentration, and eventually becomes depressed or suffers other debilitating ills—a classic passive/aggressive condition.

Even with this knowledge, some people will resist adapting reactive behavior with the defense that high-spirited action is necessary to achieve results...to get things done. Ironically, this behavior is rewarded by most organizations because it does get results over the short-term. It fails to take into account the damage done and eventually comes back to haunt them in workers compensation claims, illness, accidents, and conflicts. It is the irony of our times.

People who have figured this out have also learned that a cyclical give-and-take pattern is the best solution. No stress-free environment exists in today's modern society. So we need to be able to cope with these pressures as they occur, and to be able to release the tension that finds its way onto our physical being as a result of the stress bombardment. The release of stress often is slated for a time after the coping.

Coping is a lonely survival skill. It is not intended to be the end-all. It is temporary at best. It gives you time and freedom to prepare for the more fundamental changes in your behavior and in the external situations around you. The main coping technique around today is exercising. It helps get some of the stress off your body. Of course, it doesn't do much for other factors that strain your physical, emotional, and intellectual aspects. Ultimately the best procedure is to change your frame of mind first and then change the other things that are possible at the time and chip away at others as you can.

Taking time to look closely at yourself will give you the comfort of knowing that you already have certain abilities to begin the process in earnest. The introspective experience also helps clean away some of the debris from your personal environment.

In Deborah's case, she had a fright to get her going; she learned to handle the stress and to begin to turn her life around. If she would have had a mentor, the process would have been easier and quicker.

MENTORING: A DUTCH UNCLE

People can change by themselves once they have the process guidelines spelled out for them. A **mentor** can expedite the turn-around because of experience, wisdom, and an objective point of view. Internal change often becomes unclear to the person undergoing the shift. A mentor can offer bias-free judgment that impacts on our perceptions.

Mentoring can work two ways. You can be the mentor, or you can find one for yourself. Mentoring for someone else is usually reserved for someone who has fairly good emotional maturity but wants to polish and add a little icing to the already-baked cake. If you want to develop emotionally, recruit a mentor—someone who has the qualities you'd like to have, or at least for whose judgment you have deep respect.

Usually, the person will be someone older (although not necessarily), someone in power, and someone who is willing to take some time to assist in your development. A few organizations have formal programs, more have informal arrangements. Most have none, so you'll have to do the spadework.

The rules for mentoring vary, but all schemes generally include these four guidelines:

- expectations are agreed to out-front,

- regular meetings take place,

- all talks are confidential, and

- advice is given only when requested.

If you want to be a mentor and are asked to do so by someone in the organization, take it seriously. It means you have the qualities to be emulated and that's a good starting place for any relationship. Be direct, talk straight, and give the relationship a chance to grow.

In all cases, feelings as well as thoughts are examined in the critique of all the subsequent emotional development experiences. Being open and articulate about feelings may take some time. But don't be intimidated or tentative. Give it a try.

OVERCOMING NEGATIVES

Some love songs caution the listener to avoid falling in love because of the likelihood of having a heart broken. Without some risk—some entry into the world of feelings—a person will avoid trouble, but will miss out on most of what life offers. Living will make an old man or old woman out of you. But what's the alternative?

A mentor can help you analyze your survey scores. You'll find your scores indicate this skill or that one needs some attention. Even with scores in the Productive Zone, you'll want to study them in relation to different people and events in your life that seem a little off-key. Scores obtained are indications of your current preferences, but different people and situations may evoke a variation on theme in some cases. In those instances, you may want to adapt one, two, or more for the sake of satisfaction and productivity. When you come face to face with change, you'll also run the risk of being tentative. Here's what you can do about it.

> **Activity.** Approach this activity in a playful manner. Give yourself enough time to play around with the information from the surveys. Be as positive about the effort as you can. Some solutions may not appear as quickly as you like, but give the process time and space to work for you.
>
> Take a blank 8½ x 11 sheet of paper and draw a line vertically down the center of it so you have two equal spaces of 5½ x 8½. On the left side, write the 12 skills down the page, leaving about half an inch between each. Taking one skill at

a time, think back on the people, events and situations that currently give you trouble and list them on the opposite side of the paper. You'll probably wind up with a couple of examples for each skill—some will have more than others. By analyzing this completed page of skills and problems, you'll find an emerging plan for overcoming your tentativeness in dealing with the trouble. You'll see who and what is triggering your tentativeness and can plan accordingly.

Study each trigger and make some notes on how you can control that trigger prior to a next encounter with that person or situation. If you don't expect it to occur again, scratch it off the list. Doodle some answers, though, for those people and situations you know cause you to hesitate and act reluctantly.

When you've doodled some good first steps, take another sheet and make four columns across the page. Title one Intellectual, one Emotional, one Physical, and the fourth one Spiritual. Transpose the tentative triggers from the first page to this sheet and group them appropriately under the headings. You may have three or four under each, or more under one heading than another. All may be under the same heading—emotional problems, intellectual, physical, or spiritual. Whatever your case, you will get a graphic display that can lead you to the next step: fixing it up.

If the triggers fall equally into all four categories—intellectual, emotional, physical and spiritual—your next move is to develop strategies for each. If you find that emotional requires more work than the other three, so be it. Do this now, or do it when you are ready to begin. When you start, use the "doodle" to keep your mind sharp and yourself in soft focus. You can tighten up the first draft later when you have more comfort with the process.

CHANGING THE TRIGGERS

When you've completed the strategies for your current situation, you'll find that much of the tentativeness has mysteriously vanished, or at least you'll be willing to attempt some new behavior with people and situations that had confused or baffled you in the past. But that's only part of a synergistic solution. The next step requires both sides of your brain working together.

The test of survival is to have a vision . . .a dream . . .a hope for a better future. Your recent strategies dealt, in a reactive way, with people and events which are current in your life. Placing yourself a step beyond calls for a new model—a pattern etched of your own design and innovation. Creation of something new and stimulating can only be done by total collaboration of intellectual, emotional, and physical aspects.

> **Activity.** Take a third sheet of blank paper and draw the largest circle you can on it. Divide the circle into pie-shape quarters, and label them Intellectual, Emotional, Physical, and Spiritual. Now's a chance for you to honestly size yourself up. If you haven't done the surveys, scoring, and interpretations, you may have some difficulty here. Those who have done the work will have recent data to use for themselves.
>
> Use different colored markers, crayons, or what have you and fill up each segment to the degree of adult development you've achieved to date in your life. The part that's unfilled reveals your potential. Figure 9.9 is an example of someone who see him or herself in good physical condition, has an inquiring and inquisitive mind, and yet senses a need for emotional and spiritual maturity.

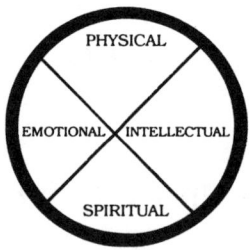

Figure 9.9. A personality model.

The parts that aren't filled in reveal your potential as you see it. This is the part that holds something new, exciting, and worthwhile for you. Use the information from the surveys and your own personal assessment of your state of affairs to determine how much growing you can and would like to do.

Save this for use when you draft your warrior's game plan later. Or take time right now to specify the positive triggers for intellectual, emotional, physical, and spiritual development.

Reading is a good intellectual trigger for self development. Kafka called a book "an axe for the frozen mind." Take a few whacks. How many different and provocative books will you read within the next three months? What disciplines will they cover? Can you learn from a book on Architecture? Zoology? Business? Poetry? History? Metaphysics? Can a browsing trip to the library occasionally, say every other Saturday, prove serendipitous? Mental stimulation, away from your normal occupational pursuits, promises quick payoffs and will help fill up the intellectual pie piece on your chart.

Spiritual development begins with listening to nature. That's what many wise and serene people say. Learn to meditate or pray. Listen and learn. Don't try to "do" things at first. Just get in touch with what God has made for you to enjoy. Nature and it's blue and green harmony are triggers for contemplation and joy. Spiritual triggers may be linked to your emotional maturity—anger, fear, hatred, and similar feelings are opportunities for higher order energies, when properly understood and directed you can become wise and bring you to serenity.

Emotional triggers can be just as rewarding. A few with which you may want to experiment are role reversal, encounter, and mentoring (discussed earlier)—all designed to help you grow to an advanced state of understanding and using feelings. A harmonious state of affairs has a logical as well as an emotional balance to it. Men are especially susceptible to be out of balance in favor of logic—such is our culture today. Many women have been socialized to use their intuitive and emotional side, while men have been brought up to depend more on left brain skills. (Writer Carlos Casteneda believed that this socialization makes women better candidates than men for crusadership.) Anything less than close balance between your ability to use the two sides of the brain puts the individual in a less than efficient posture. We looked at role reversal earlier, now let's look at encounters.

Encounters are a little more touchy and may require a third party to coordinate and mediate. Try one on your own first, though.

> **Activity.** Find an issue that is in conflict with one of your core values. Maybe someone doubts or challenges your competence in technical or people terms. Or it may be your lack of involvement or too much drive, so that you seem to be interrupting the process. Or you aren't seen as a team player. Or you tell it like it is with little regard for consequences. Whatever the criticism, and wherever it comes from, accept it as valid in this instance.
>
> Face off with the person, who is critical of you, for a specific amount of time, say 20 minutes. Take the first five minutes for the two of you to define your terms and air out your feelings. Then discuss the issue openly. Give the other party equal air time. Stop after 20 minutes and critique the experience.
>
> Calm down and assess all aspects of the encounter. If you have access to a video tape recorder, record the encounter and then playback the recording so as to critique the experience from two levels, content and process—rational and intuitive. A third party can be helpful in this assessment, especially in the beginning and particularly when a sensitive topic has been the bases of the encounter. Dr. Dan Dana of Bloomfield, Ct., formerly of the University of Hartford, has developed a video-assisted mediation format that all supervisors in organizations can use to learn this conflict resolution technique quickly and under very professional guidance. Another step in the crusader process.

At some point in time, you may want to join an encounter group for further development in learning how to discipline your emotions. Know for what you're looking before joining one. Ask around. Many different ones exist. Some have drop-in formats so you can check them out before signing on. Don't be intimidated or tentative. These behaviors are signs of emotional immaturity.

For the **physical development,** you may want to drop a few pounds, quit smoking, firm up a little, take up jogging or biking on a regular basis, and try any of the zillion other diet/nutrition, exercise and relaxation techniques around today. Breaking a sweat through some rigorous but well-thought-out program will go a long way to develop your stamina and strength and keep you fit to reach the development stage you want. The statistics for good health are mainly physically-based, and fitness correlates with peak performance over the long term.

If you're a gregarious person, you may want to work out with others. Even loners find this helpful to keep them going. Once you've established a pattern, you'll find that you need to keep finding new triggers to continue the interest. The mere setting of goals frequently isn't enough, especially if you have a lot of weight to lose or a long-standing habit to break. The key is to make the process exciting enough to carry you to completion.

COMBINE YOUR NEEDS TO CREATE SYNERGY

If you decide that your diet and nutritional state of affairs is not what it should be in a life of fast-food stores and Snack City, pick up a book on nutrition. Or read one of the many health publications in the library—or at your news stand—or go to a specialist in nutrition and have an analysis done. Learn more about the seven food groups, not just the four that you grew up learning about. Here's a mini-lesson:

1. **Water** is the only genuine body fluid need. Eight glasses a day quenches your thirst for water. Fruit juices, milk, tea, alcohol, coffee, et cetera, are not body fluid needs; they are choices.

2. **Carbohydrates,** such as starches and sugars, (potatoes and apples, respectively, are examples) must be eaten whole to extract the energy needed for the rest of the bodily functions. Processed foods don't count as much, because they are so depleted.

3. **Ten amino acids** are essential to sustain life and must be taken together to produce the protein we need. Taking five for lunch and five for dinner will not do the trick. Ten together. You get them by eating from the seven groups and knowing how the combination fits together. A visit with a good nutritionalist is in order.

4. **Fats** and **oils** get a lot of attention on T.V. and in weight loss clinics, but they are essential for cellular structure and metabolism. They may not look good as fat deposits, but we need 'em. There is good cholesterol and bad. Find out which is best for your health.

5. **Vitamins** play an important role in how we put all the rest of our food input to good use. They are biochemical catalysts for cellular metabolism. You may need to supplement your diet with pills, or you may not—depends on your diet.

6. **Minerals** come in two nutrient groups, one of which we need in large amount: calcium, magnesium, potassium, sodium, phosphorus, and chlorine. Of the remaining 14, we require only micro amounts. Don't tamper with supplements—as they can be toxic—unless you have it on good authority. Discover your personal need and eat those foods which provide the proper amounts.

7. Foods that provide **pectin, fiber, cellulose,** and **mucins** are the last need—bulk. These are essential for proper gastro-intestinal and bowel functions. Use those that fit your lifestyle and that you enjoy—vegetables and some cereals fill the bill.

If you embark on a nutritional program, learn more about vegetables, meat and poultry, dairy products, fruits, nuts, grains and, of course, supplements. Look at yourself as a "corporation" or system. Through the discovery process, you'll find resources to keep you healthy. (This lesson serves as a starting place. The library, your health professional, and other resources are available for more detailed and personalized assistance.)

Take some time now and draft your new triggers for intellectual, emotional, physical, and spiritual development. Use the trigger outline described earlier, or be creative and come up with your own format. You'll soon see that development in one sector influences your perception and improvement of other sectors. Of course some overlap exists to be sure. They are interconnected. We know that and so will you as you develop your strategies for success.

THE WRONG PATH

If intimidation and tentativeness are enemies to starting the crusade to finding yourself, then false lures and sidetracks are serious pitfalls. Everyone has their own false lures, but these following examples will clarify these terms. (These are based on real experiences.)

John S. parlayed high energy, a quick wit, and a sense of numbers into a budding career as a financial planning consultant after paying his dues with one of the Big Eight accounting firms. Success took the usual material form of a big, well-furnished house, two cars, the club membership, a time-share vacation condo and, of course, designer clothes for himself and his wife. At age 38, John S. couldn't do anything but get better, except for two character flaws . . .women and booze.

He was not what you'd call Hollywood handsome but more like the guy next door, with well-kept good looks. John had always liked girls when growing up and, even though he had experienced some trouble expressing himself to them, he figured he'd outgrow that dilemma. Drinking, on the other hand, had never been a problem. He liked to drink, could handle it, and drank a lot and often. The combination proved to be nearly fatal.

To perk himself up after an exceptionally disappointing day, John stopped at a new hotel bar, recently renovated and rumored to be a "body shop" for divorced and mature singles. As he sat at the bar and scanned the crowd, he mused his approval. The room was quiet—quieter than most singles hangouts anyway—and the people had an allure that struck him. After two drinks, he made eye contact and asked Cindi to join him. One thing led to another and, over the next three years, John repeated this and similar scenes. His wife finally gave up and filed for divorce. John still doesn't know why he stopped growing and followed the path of least resistance to a painful, personal defeat.

Unable or unwilling to face up to small defeats in business, John turned from making minor corrections in his business tactics to the lure of conquest. Drinking made him feel better emotionally—a temporary condition—and a deep-seated drive to make up for those early years of discomfort with females put him in situations where he had to prove himself time and again. The lure of emotional stability out-weighed his business stability, which seemed trifling at the moment. One little setback seemed too trivial to pursue. The inner ache didn't.

A counselor would likely have told John to get on with correcting the flaws in his business plan and work through those difficulties first before addressing the drinking and womanizing issues. Once his self-esteem, in a business sense, had been cleaned up, John could have learned that most young boys and men have difficult times with emotional expression, heightened by members of the opposite sex.

His philandering proved to be a substitute for getting on with it. Once this became apparent, John would have been on his way. Knowing, by itself, can cure the lure on some occasions. As in fishing, the false lure can be destructive if you're the fish. In Oriental philosophy, the net and the fish work together. In John's case, mentor, a friend, or a counselor could have been beneficial. His company didn't provide one and he didn't ask for help.

A WAY OF LIFE FOR THE SIDETRACKER

Sidetracking, though, is a different than straight talk and more complex than ordinary technical problems. Again, the example is real.

Straight Talk and Side Track have the same initials, but the similarity ends there. Examine this dialogue and get the sense of these differences. The Straight Talker is Jean, the Sidetracker is Jane.

> Jean: *My gosh, it's been two, no, three years since I've seen you. How's Ted and the kids?*
>
> Jane: *It hasn't been three years. It couldn't have been. I remember seeing you at Albertson's market a few months ago. I tried to get your attention, though. You hurried off and I had a list as long as my arm. My, time does fly, doesn't it. How's Rick doing in his new job?*
>
> Jean: *Rick's been promoted and we'll be moving to Atlanta next month when the kids are out of school. I suppose—*
>
> Jane: (interrupting) *Isn't that just like big companies. Just when you've gotten settled in here they go and move you off to some deserted island or someplace like that. I just can't understand it. It's why I'm glad Ted decided—with my help, of course—to stay with my father's insurance business. No Atlanta for us, No Sirree.*
>
> Jean: *Well, I've got to run, Jane. Nice seeing you again.*

Sidetrackers generally have two distinct characteristics. One is they can't seem to focus on what's happening in the here and now. The other, and probably more damning, is the inability to manage their time. They also find themselves engrossed in multiples. They hop and skip from one thing to another, never gaining closure on one. With more balls in the air than even the most expert juggler would attempt, the sidetracker goes blisslessly on his or her way to nowhere.

Sidetracking is often a symptom of "burnout," a psycho-emotional condition of drained human energies. By being too intense for too long a time, these individuals suddenly are out of gas. Their instincts tell them to continue going, but the

mental computer fails to function as it once did. They work in gray colors—wandering from point to point, often not remembering where they are going and what they're supposed to do once they arrive.

When involved in confrontation or even casual conversation, they can't seem to quite nail down the point. They drift a lot. By looking at the Sphere of Influence Cone (Figure 9.10) on a personal level, you can see how sidetracks can cost you.

Life's Issues

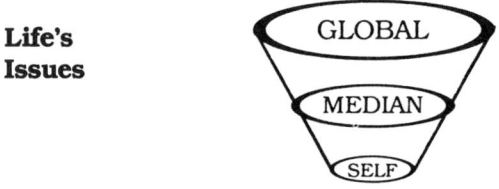

Figure 9.10. Sphere of influence cone .

The cone emphasizes your personal issues at three distinct levels—global, median, and personal. A global issue is something like poverty, famine, or war. The counterparts in median issues would be the economic status in your neighborhood, a wheat crop failure in your state, and the family argument next door. Personal issues in the same vein would be when you and your spouse go broke, you go to the bare cupboard, and you are mugged on a dark street.

While these descriptors may be negative, they do explain the degree of difference of some real issues facing people today. Take poverty. A few people may be able to address that global issue, the United Nations Assembly might, or key leaders in government. Not many just plain folks, though, will impact or influence this issue without spending a lot of time and energy to marshal resources for a global assault.

On the other hand, if the issue was on the most personal or self level, they could do something about it. They can find a solution, get a job, take a hand-out. Or they could starve to death, a form of suicide.

In a previous anecdote, John S. did not commit suicide, but he did grievous damage to himself and his family. A self issue is generally in complete control of the individual. It's where your influence is at its greatest and can bring about the most immediate result.

Imagine the bottom circle in the cone representing your wish to stop smoking. . .or drinking. . . or doing drugs. Once you decide to do so, it's completely within your reach to achieve the goal. You take the time and energy to adapt your behavior. Even if you go to a professional clinic to get assistance, it's still your decision and your action.

If you were to fill in the self circle completely when you changed the behavior, you'd have the satisfaction of winning. Fill in the same sized circle in the median circle and you would leave a large void to be filled. The void represents the amount of frustration you'd suffer. Move the self circle to the global level and you find even less satisfaction and more frustration. The key is to stay within that part of the cone which offers the best chance for winning. At this stage of the adaptation process, it's at the self level. Later, when projects are established for changing group lifestyles, and corporate lifestyles, you'll see how to move up the cone with strategies directed at larger issues.

To address median and global issues requires planning. You need to get others involved in drafting non-smoking legislation, publicizing the harmful effects of smoking, and the like. Without such support, you'll burn out.

Once you've made the commitment to stop abusing, to lose weight, or stop being defensive about this or that, you can change your behavior in a relatively short span of time, with a good plan and some support. When you start to move up the cone, though, and attempt to influence others to do what you want them to do, it becomes much more complex, and time and energy consuming.

If you feel you have sidetracking tendencies, do what the survivors do. Lay some solid track for yourself. Try it on your own first. The situation may only be a temporary condition, sparked by a sudden turn of events or a series of mishaps. You need to pull it out of yourself. No one did it to you, so no one is going to do it for you. Follow the guidelines written here.

If you wish, get some help. If family or friends are incapable, or seem so, go to a professional counselor for a short spell. Remember, though, that the last thing you need is another crutch.

Once on track, do what good baseball teams do. . .get an insurance run. A habit is only a good one if you can do it without thinking. The instincts are there for Straight Talk, but it takes practice.

> **Activity for Straight Talk.** Talk to children as a test. Don't talk as a parent or Big Person but as an innocent. Get on their level, on the floor, and listen to them and their questions.
>
> Be in touch with your emotions as you do this. Listen to yourself as you listen to them. Listen at both levels to everyone. Meditate on solutions. Keep track of the content and the process. It won't always be possible to do it perfectly. So what? Keep trying. It will become first nature, once again. Like when you were a kid.

SUMMARY

Those who have survival skills and value success can be models for those who are in the process of developing their own.

Experts, like Toffler, point to the individual as the key to survival in this crazy, mixed-up world of ours. The better your balance, the better chance for surviving.

The triggers we've discussed can either toss or energize you. Without a plan, you'll tend to react to people and events, lessening your chance for success. Try the systems approach, do like Deborah Elkin did as discussed in this chapter, do as the role model of your choice did, or find a mentor. Do your homework. Research your health and performance need.

Replace poor behaviors with the positiveness of your choice.

Stay in the bottom of the cone until you're ready for full scale combat. Live neoteny. Stay youthful with the world. Stay mentally alert, physically vigorous, emotionally balanced, and spiritually accessible.

Do the Surveys and activities now if you haven't already done them.

CHAPTER **10**

CAPTURE THE MOMENT

The music filled the room like a cloud of tulle fog rolling across a valley, moving in slowly, swirling white/grey wisps. For a five-year-old, Tommy Ward had unusual tastes in records. **"The kid's as eclectic as a late night radio station disc jockey,"** *his father would joke to friends.* **"I don't know where he gets his taste,"** *he'd invariably add.*

A recent favorite song, **"You Belong to the City,"** *filtered softly through the speakers as Tommy worked a piece of the complex Transformer toy system, making first a robot and then a race car of sleek and realistic proportions. His young mind was completely absorbed with what his hands were doing, yet his eyes sparkled almost in tune to the music. Here, in this little boy's bedroom, magic was at work. Tommy Ward was in a state of euphoric ecstasy—the wisdom and serenity model in action.*

His parents didn't understand the mystery of their boy's talent to **"lose himself"** *in what he was doing. Tommy, with the help of music, could connect his being to another dimension—a synergistic capturing of his physical, intellectual, emotional, and spiritual facets.*

Their friends all made pointed comments to his **"precociousness,"** *or to his being* **"exceptional"** *but Walt and Ellen didn't realize the extent of his potential. Nor did they understand, at this stage in his development, their responsibility to nurture its growth.*

Maybe if they had other, more normal children, the lustre of this son would have caught their attention. Or if they had been less involved in their own uncertainties, it would have been more apparent. They probably would have witnessed his depth had they not been so caught up in valium and cocktails every evening.

INTRODUCING THE PLANNING PROCESS

Some parents have the belief that children are brought into being as a kind of old-age insurance policy, guarding against their frailty—someone to care for them when they've become invalid or disabled. Others, like many you see at Little League and Little Theater, believe that children are an opportunity to live the life they missed for one reason or another. Only a handful of parents in this country, according to information found in doing research for this book, are aware of the idea that every member of the family has unique talents and special needs of their own.

In a very few fortunate situations, the needs merge and the talents can be reflected in common endeavors. The following folk tale may give you an idea of why knowing this is important for your personal, team, and family success.

The Ashanti Tribe in Africa recall the Tale of Anansi, the Spider. Anansi is the proud father of six children, each of whom develops a distinctive skill suited to the young spider's abilities. They frolic and play and generally enjoy life growing up in a happy and cared-for environment.

One day Anansi travels far from their village and tumbles into some serious trouble. He falls into a deep ravine and is caught in a mesh of bramble from which he's unable to free himself.

The children are hard at play as night approaches, and suddenly they begin to worry about Father. One son, known as Signal Catcher because of his ability to listen so well, listens hard and picks up the sound waves being sent by the trapped Anansi. They huddle around another child, known as Road Maker, who maps out the way they will take to find Father.

Following Road Maker for a spell, they come upon a large pond which stands in their way and prevents further advancement toward their stricken relative. A third child, called Water Drinker, puts that skill to work and drains the pond so they can continue the rescue mission.

After more frenetic charging ahead, they suddenly see before them a huge crevasse. They are dismayed. There's no way to get across an opening so wide until the fourth child, known as Chasm Spanner, puts that skill to the test and builds a bridge over the huge opening.

Darkness falls and they begin to wander from the path set by Road Maker. It's getting so dark they can't possibly continue. Chaos appears to have caught up with the search party until the bright child, called Light the Way, steps forward to keep the six going forward with the fire-fly ability.

At last they come to the fateful place where Anansi has fallen, and they see he is well out of their reach, caught in the brambles. All hope is about given up when the sixth child steps forward and demonstrates her skill. She is called Rope Maker.

Later, back in the village, the celebrating continues all day. Anansi is pleased with his children's collaboration, and all seems well until bickering breaks out, each child proclaiming his or her skill the most important in the rescue of Father. Anansi, who wishes to reward them, calls upon God for assistance to quell the bickering and for a way to show his pleasure to all of them.

The Ashanti God tells Anansi to poll the family to determine what memorial each would find pleasurable for taking part in the rescue. Anansi does and returns to God with this description: It must be beautiful, it must have utility, and, **above all, it must be enduring. Having heard Anansi, God shows him a huge, white, glowing globe and asks,** *"Like this?"*

"Oh, yes," answers an awed Anansi. *"That's exactly what they desire."* Hearing the words, God hurls the object into the dark night towards the sky, saying, *"It will remain there night after night for all to see."*

Whether you receive a moon or a star as your memorial for doing your part in caring for those in trouble at home or at work, it's good to know that teamwork and risk taking are valued commodities. The inevitable bickering over whose skill is more valued will subside when the rewards are seen to be just and equal. The Tale does highlight the notion that skills development is critical, each in its own way useful to the process. As an example of synergy, what also is pointed out is that some time is needed to make the process work—a disciplined participation.

THE ART OF DISCIPLINED PARTICIPATION

One school that practices the lesson of disciplined participation is James Logan High School (JLHS). Located in a tough, gritty part of the East Bay between San Francisco and San Jose, Logan was recently awarded "exemplary status," one of 63 schools in the nation to be so designated by President Ronald reagan. Principal Jim O'Laughlin of the Union City, California, school believes in the "total learning" concept. He is also a realist.

His school went from a 39% minority base to 61% in ten years in an old but growing urban community impacted by an influx of immigrants and refugees. About 30% of the 2,640 students come from low-income families and 12% have English as a second language, speaking it with varying degrees of fluency. The parents, of course, don't speak it at all. *"The key to helping educate this population is to clarify the expectations of everyone concerned,"* O'Laughlin began the explanation.

O'Laughlin follows simple but inflexible guidelines in running a tight ship. He closed the campus to ward off drug dealers as much as possible. Classroom doors are closed when the bell rings and students can't get in without an approved pass.

"Teachers get 50 minutes without interruption to teach every class. You can't learn skills if you're not in class or come in late and cause a disruption for others," he elucidates.

With guidelines in place, people began showing up on time. The best part is that each course has been revamped to be suitable to the make-up of the school's population. It was part of a plan and it was working.

Seven years ago the decision was made to do something more about the plight of education at the school. The realization that "teaching" is not a 9-to-5 job sunk in. Jim O'Laughlin and his predecessor took a strident stance towards marshalling the forces needed to mount an assault on community apathy, political inertia, and the assorted non-interest groups ranging from students to teachers. They stopped and looked around and decided they needed a plan. They wound up with a systems approach. It has several distinct components that connect synergistically to each other and it is evolving to meet changing needs. The major reason it flourishes is because of widespread and convincing support.

The support group includes parents, the community, the funding sources, the local administration, the teachers, and, to a solid extent, the kids themselves. Teachers and administrators play pivotal roles, of course. They take a part of each year to go over the plan for the coming year. *"It generally means more hours out front, but it pays back dividends by the time graduation rolls around,"* O'Laughlin added. And, being multi-faceted, it includes real measurement. Teachers are observed by peers and administrators and they also grade themselves. Evaluation addresses and deals with incompetency, O'Laughlin pointed out, bucking a system that usually protects all, even the incompetent.

Outstanding teachers may get special assignments, working on projects in the school to broaden their skills base in the classroom. The school is run like a business and it has measurable Bottom Lines. This planning and evaluation approach earned top grades in the nation despite economic deprivation—countering the age-old argument that good education means higher costs.

O'Laughlin believes children can benefit from an even earlier start at balancing their total development to reach their potential, supporting the mentoring work being done by Louis Lerman across the Bay in wealthy Palo Alto, on the same campus that finds American conservatism in full flower.

INVESTING IN CHILDREN

Louis Lerman, a Hertz Fellow at Stanford University, is a scientist by training and innovator by inclination. Lerman believes Silicon Valley and other centers of high technology not only should attract the brightest, most creative thinkers of our time, but he feels they should support research and development of young people. Until he sells that concept, Lerman is acting on his belief and is conducting a science education experiment on his own.

For two hours a week, Lerman works with ten children, ages eight to ten, and serves as a mentor to develop their total brain—left and right sides. Lerman encourages exploration and experimentation so the young people can see and understand what they perceive. They use the facilities at Stanford to the fullest and the result is that the kids gain confidence in themselves so they can amplify their own impulses for discovery.

The exhilaration that comes from discovery, according to Lerman, is common to all of us and is something we never lose. Some, he notes, give up their willingness to try or trust their own perceptions. His systems approach fosters self-confidence and independence of thought and action. He's teaching soft focus and the kids are learning to stay in balance while they achieve.

Lerman's kids do projects well beyond their years. They began writing educational programs based on their experiences in Basic, a primary computer language, found it too restrictive, and now are taking on the more complicated but structured Pascal programming language. Talk has even occurred about starting their own software company and marketing their products to other kids their own age.

What Lerman has discovered is that the traditional school doesn't offer the challenge and opportunity a curious child needs to stimulate both sides of the brain. His experiments, although limited, are noteworthy enough to focus attention on what might be a stake in this country's future educational effectiveness. It might be fun, too.

HOPE RISES AND EXPECTATIONS GROW

State and federal governments can offer more support for bridging education to the world of work. If people are to spend 20, 30, and often more, years in a productive capacity, the schools must do their share in readying young America for the struggle. Common skills will no longer suffice in a changing, complex society.

James Logan HS, replete with two, and soon to be three computer labs, mostly earned through community funding projects co-chaired by teachers, students, parents, and business people, goes against the grain, as most winners do. Textbooks have a role in the process, but not at the expense of emotional education. JLHS takes a cue from Ned Herrmann's GE research and works both sides of the brain, skilling all involved with as much responsibility for success as they can absorb.

While Herrmann attempts to recoup lost opportunities through art and creativity training, JLHS models the balance in basic values and total lifestyle skills which enables its graduates to seek out opportunities that likely will not echo their initial economic deprivation. All at JLHS share their expectations our front and live life to meet them. They're a step ahead right now. It's called preparation—a vital step in changing corporate lifestyles. if such synergy can work in a high school, it surely can find a home where you work.

IBM, for example, requires its managers to partake of 60 hours of professional education each year, including 24 hours on the "people" side. This is up from 40 hours only a few years ago, of which 36 were spent on the technology of the business. Big Blue has learned that technology is part of the game, but that the softer skills are becoming important as the struggle for supremacy heats up.

By allocating 3.75% of the manager's available time at work for rational and intuitive education—both left and right brain—IBM virtually assures itself dominance in its field...at least until its competitors pick up on the practice.

Even though IBM's approach continues to be imbalanced in favor of technology, the new distribution of time for learning is progress in the right direction.

That's what's going on at the leader. What's your company doing? What percentage of the 1600 working hours a year does your company invest in your future, and its own?

Whatever the answer is, a good idea might be to listen to what *Business Week* wrote a while back, quoting Bill Crockett, former chief of staff to Dean Rusk at the State Department and most recently head of human resources at Saga Foods. Bill said it might be time to just stop all training and education and simply find out what the real needs of the organization are—disciplined participation.

Bill and others in his field find that so much of what's passed off as training and development is really ego-stroking and fad. He noted that not too much difference occurs whether in the private or the public sector. Neither is following a systems approach and a good assumption may be that most training efforts are probably causing more damage than good, especially when all the costs are added up.

Current training and development, interestingly enough, may be adding to your health care bill. People taking time off to attend valueless classes and courses possibly will get sick from them. It's undisciplined. The anxiety of being off the job and not getting something out of the time is a costly experience, adding to an already stressful psyche.

Participants may enjoy being entertained initially, but when they are unable to implement esoteric bits of fad or fluff, they tend to have an anxiety attack. Nothing has changed back at the work station, the paper has stacked up, the boss continues to pressure for "more" and the dreaded Status Quo fails to respond to the non-directed attempt at education.

The trend of "lecture series" featuring well-oiled talkers, some with impressive credentials, others with mainly a glib presentation designed to entertain, is a poor excuse for providing people with a key to unlock the synergism stored inside them. On a corporate level, the operating system, which works directly from the strategic plan will enable people to grow and fulfill themselves, while meeting the expectations of the employer.

LISTENING TO THE MESSAGE

Whether or not you are predisposed to someone or not, the crusader knows he or she can learn by active listening, which means getting something out of the information that you can use for personal growth and development. On a higher level—the spiritual level—you learn best by going deeper within yourself.

Near the end of writer/actress Shirley MacLaine's book, *Don't Fall Off the Mountain*, she tells of reframing her values after being exposed to the poverty and desolation in Calcutta, India. What she meant was, after such a deeply moving and touching experience, she reordered her core values so a new, more appropriate energy and direction took place in her life.

Tommy Ward's parents could have experienced a similarly moving and touching experience had they been more focused and sober to the moment of their son's capability. Any parent can. The core values are designed to meet this change in motivation and become a part of it. Figure 10.1 is an example of a typical person's values and their intensity—satisfaction/frustration ratio.

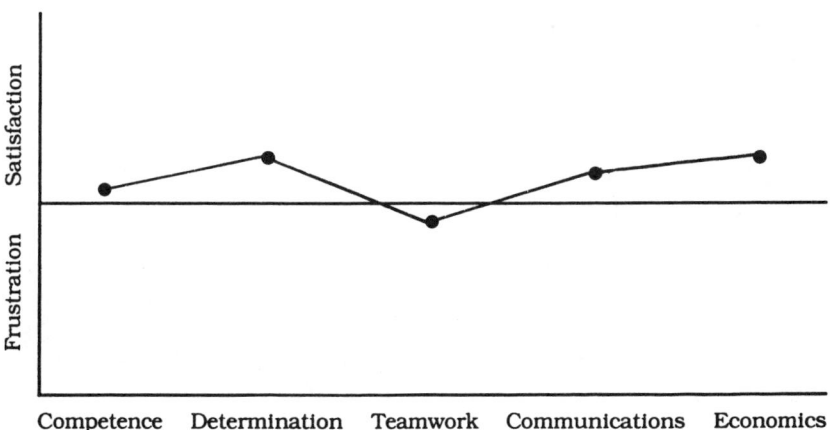

Figure 10.1. Core value profile.

Like the LED dial on a high tech stereo system, the chart points out the highs and low of your motivational energy—the driving force for action. Highs for this personalized example illustrate good satisfaction from Economics with a modicum of emotional spark from Competence and Determination, but a low output from Teamwork and Communications.

In a work situation, this could be someone who is well-paid, is using talents to produce quality output, but is frustrated with others in the work group and with how information or feedback is given. If this profile was taken at home, the person would be pleased with the budget, probably even accumulating wealth through investments and savings. He or she may have a hobby to keep competencies going and is satisfied about that outcome, but registers disappointment on the values of Teamwork and communications, which means not every one is pulling their weight, and no real dialogue is taking place. The "Where you been?" "Out." syndrome.

To follow Shirley MacLaine's lead, each individual would have to reframe his or her values to be much more Teamwork and Communications-minded. Doing so would not necessarily mean making less money or saving less; not at all. In the reframing process, you can develop new energies through development of your spiritual self. It may take you away from the Economics orientation without losing a thing materially. In some cases, one could wind up in making less, but enjoying life more.

The important thing to know is that a revitalized spirit can produce higher levels of motivation for the overlooked or undermined values of family and intimacy through sharing—a criterion for healthy communications with loved ones.

Young people, like a Tommy Ward, can "capture the moment" easier that a lot of adults. They can listen to music, work with their hands, free their minds, and pull everything all together so that they enjoy to the fullest whatever they happen to be engaged in at that instant in time. Music helps.

THE BEAT OF A DIFFERENT DRUMMER

A game of developing some higher sense of yourself comes from listening to the harmonics of life, which is often portrayed in song. Music has been a part of this civilization and previous ones. The drum was animal skin pulled over a hollowed log; the river reed became a flute; slivers of metal stretched across a gourd became a guitar. Children grasp this readily. They know the lyrics to countless songs to which some parents swear the words are unintelligible.

Activity

The game is simple. Get a pad of paper, a pen or pencil and set aside some listening time over a period of a week or two. Play one or two songs from the following categories:

GOSPEL ROCK JAZZ COUNTRY POPULAR SWING BLUES

After getting comfortable, play the song(s) from one category and write your reactions on the paper. Listen with your eyes closed on one set and with them open on another. Write in stream of consciousness format. When you've gone through two or three categories, analyze what you've written from the standpoint of emotional and spiritual content, forgetting somewhat how you reacted physically or intellectually.

With a focus on feelings and spirit, you'll discover a deeper aspect of your listening ability. You'll also find a subtle but important difference from what you felt with eyes open or closed. Imagery tends to be better when you close your eyes—we're a very visually-oriented and eye-dependent culture. If you don't experience any differences, you may alread be well-attuned. Or, you may not be experiencing the sounds well enough. You're the best judge of what's happening.

Adolescents performing this activity find the next step intriguing. And that is to write a spiritual description of songs from each category. They stretch their development by putting down on paper words—poems or prose—to what occurs to their mood when taking a more active part in the harmony drill.

CAN SCHOOLS CHANGE?

William C. Bennett, secretary of education in the Reagan Administration, is a crusader. He came by it naturally; his parents practiced as well as preached spiritual strengthening. When he advocated changes in schools, it came from experience as well. Training in law as well as school administration, he brought a strong background in the arts to the job. Bennett served as head of the National Endowment for the Arts Foundation before taking the top educational post in the land. People tend to combine what they know with what they have to do.

Bennett knew that educators like O'Laughlin and Lerman are the exceptions, not the rule in this country today. He knew that four things must happen before the educational process is maximized in this country: Parents, teachers, principals and students must all work in harmony.

Parents, Bennett told the Parent/Teachers Association recently, must be more involved in education, especially in the home. Parents, too, can exert more pressure on school boards to set agendas, but spending more time in creating an appreciation and skills in the arts will be a major progression.

Teachers, too, have a responsibility to be more professional and accept the idea of performance evaluation before demanding more pay. In-service training, as currently constituted, may not be nearly effective enough to cope with changing and complex needs of the country.

Principals, Bennett believed, are the critical part of the process. "If you only have time and money enough for one condition, focus on the principal," he told the group. A good principal is like the owner of a Mom-Pop grocery store in the bygone years. They know where everything and everyone is and what it takes to make ends meet. The good principal is a professional manager with the added talent of probably having spent time as a parent and teacher, although neither is necessarily a requirement.

Students, of course, play an important part. They can disrupt the process by acting up or laying down on the job. If they get excited early on about learning, though, they're a joy to be with. Children need to know the expectations and the rules of the school. One third grade class Bennett talked about knew the rules: "No messing around, no fooling around, no mistakes and everybody loves you." A pretty good description for an exemplary school in any part of the country. The best part of it is that it doesn't take any more money to run a good school than it does a poor one.

THE SPIRITUALITY ASPECT

Looking at people at work, and parents in their homes, the problems they have stem probably from a long-time-ago trigger. The fact is that most adult problems with drugs, booze, relationship, and the like are linked to adolescence. The missing link in that chain from young to old is spirituality. The universal energy that helps create a more satisfying frame for the core values—a display case—comes from connecting to a higher order of yourself.

You don't necessarily have to go to church or bend your knees to acquire the power to crusade and change your situation. In most cases, doing so doesn't hurt your chances. The point is that you can do both. The once-a-week tribute to spiritual development simply isn't enough. A little more time is needed so you can spend even more time being on a higher plane—what Eric Berne called Intimacy.

Shirley MacLaine's interest in yoga followed her revelations in India. This meditative way to liberate your spirit is well-founded. Any meditation and calming down of our anxieties is useful. it will also allow us to get in touch with the inner and more quiet energy that exists and lays dormant.

Whether you listen to music, meditate, pray, or simply "be" with nature, you'll, at least, renew yourself, and, at best, get in touch with a potential power that's yours for the taking.

SUMMARY

Music, so the saying goes, soothes the savage beast. It also soothes the internal beast.

Education is complemented by appreciation of music and other art forms.

Parents and children can play together and harmonize their lives.

Creativity is generally stifled going through the institutions of learning. This can be corrected by crusading parents. For the sake of their young.

CHAPTER **11**

STRETCHING THE PROCESS

The little boy tugged at his mother's skirt as they walked down the aisle of the fancy department store: **"Mommy, I gotta potty."**

"Honey, you just went before we got here!" Tommy Ward's mother tried to reason with him.

"I know, Mommy. But I gotta go again," he reasoned back.

The two-year-old generally got his way. He was the delight of his mother's life, and only once in a while did his father object to the attention. Both parents adored the boy, especially because he came so late in their lives.

Little Tommy changed their lives dramatically and they didn't realize it at first. Accustomed to eating out frequently, joining their friends for long weekends, and doing what young couples without the burden of toddlers generally do. A conservatism crept into their lives and slowly but steadily darkened their own, personal outlook—without them realizing it.

The boy was a dream come true—he was strong, healthy, bright, and appealing. Strangers stopped Ellen on the street to comment on his attractiveness.

Oblivious to all the consternation, Tommy Ward smiled as his mother pulled up his pants in the restroom. **"Thanks, Mommy. We go shoppin'?"** *Tommy, age 2, kept track of where he was.*

MAKING EACH MOVE COUNT

Developing a collaborative rather than a competitive work environment has a chance for success today because people want it for their own health, while the corporation welcomes the economic fruits of healthy new lifestyles. further supporting the work-smoothly-together movement is the practice of measuring gains and losses both on a personal and corporate level. The theory being that the better you play the game, the more likely you are to register the win.

Unfortunately, the most common form of measurement in most organization is simply win/lose. The idea of "how you play the game" has some backers, but in the main, who comes out on top in the short run is what counts. Then, too, this competitive nature is carried back home, where a family habit of put-downs becomes destructive, albeit it's all done with a smile on face. A synergistic transplant would be helpful.

Evaluation has lived a precarious life in the corporation despite a wealth of money being spent on it and countless hours of form-filling around descriptive ratios, targets, stretch goals, and objectives. It is a cold-hearted process that could benefit from an injection of humanity..a little fuel for the fading fire.

The business place and its many formats, MBO (management by objectives, or in some cases by objection), MBI (management by innuendo), MBR (management by results or rationality), and similar acronyms have been too inconsistent to be taken seriously any longer. Only rarely has the business place or one of its formats produced the self-arousal necessary for people to make commitments to the place where they work.

As more senior executives become familiar with concepts expanding the traditional, technical, and left-brain orientation, the likelihood that synergy will flourish increases. With acceptance will come practice. Practice will change the corporate lifestyle and improve the facility to measure it. Life styles lend themselves to clearcut evaluation at the personal, work group, and corporate levels in the organization. The also can be evaluated at home and throughout society. Support for this premise is building momentum and includes a formidable group of advocates. Motivational theorists aside, employee-sensitive, project-dominated measurement looms on the horizon.

The biggest problem with current employee appraisals is the subjectivity of them—a right brain phenomenon. One man's meat will always be another's poison. Few of us see the same event in the same light and the differences in perception have clouded the face-to-face confrontations that so many supervisors dread.

Many managers are not harmonious enough with their subordinates to give them useful feedback. Survey respondents are unequivocal in their distaste for current evaluation programs. They see them as punishment. Those willing to change like the idea, though, of a values-based system that would give balance, first, and allow for easy and direct talk to teammates, second. Genuine excitement over such a system that puts harmony into projects and evaluation can be felt in quiet talks about what's possible to do around here.

KEEP HOME FIRES BURNING AND BURNING

Evaluation is critical to maintain high levels of performance. Without a "pay for performance" plan of some sort, people will not generate the energy needed to spark the organization's engines. Money helps close the process. such closure is essential for all concerned. Without a close, energy tends to dwindle and drip away. Engineers call it line loss.

That's what keeps students trying so hard to stay on honor rolls and the dean's list. It's what inspires most professional athletes to outperform last year's standards. it's what keeps the artist at the canvas or whittling at large chunks of shapeless metal, ceramic, and wood. Most professionals at work, however, have been deprived of such feedback. The feedback at home, at best, is questionable. Unlike Tommy Ward, who knew where he was and what he wanted to do, many of us are left wondering.

We dote on the win/lose phenomenon and regret its prevalence in work and at home. We play hurtful games rather than focus on supportive team behaviors. Most professionals have heard of the win/win proposition, but only in passing. Some equate it to a "dead heat" in a horse race, not a common happening. Not very many have felt it personally. A win/win phenomenon is really a performance index in which all the players know the scoring system—a melding of content and process.

It's been hailed and embraced in those few places where it's been properly implemented and maintained.

THE UNIVERSAL MEASUREMENT

The win/win performance index can be tailored to any organization. It can be developed for a hospital, government agency, educational unit, human services office, retail store, transportation company, bank or other financial institution, high tech enterprise, manufacturing firm, public utility, or a group of lawyers. It is best done by those involved in the operation of the business. It works for the family, too.

Whether you're in the business of goods or services or both, the people doing the work have the best knowledge available—what they lack is a structure that makes sense. The manager can facilitate this process with a structure to generate ideas, and then put them into project form, complete with a values-based scoring system. That's what happened at Johns Hopkins Medical Institute in Baltimore, Maryland. (Names will be omitted here to protect the sensitivity of the situation.)

A new administrator arrived on the scene at one of the research and teaching departments and felt a need to find out as much as possible about the competencies of the people as quickly as he could. The administrator called on the human resource specialist for help and was offered five programs to facilitate the "getting to know people" process.

Instinctively, the administrator selected the Synergy System. The name intrigued him, the price was right, and it could be installed with little muss and fuss. The 25 staff members were informed of these intentions and began working on self assessments, followed by group activities, and eventually concluded with a plan that included an evaluation index of budget, treatment, caseloads, therapies, and time ratios.

The administrator was gratified. Getting to know who was willing to live up to the expectations, and more, was fruitful. One initially reluctant manager disclosed that ". . . going to strengths rather than trying to shore up weaknesses enabled the staff to upgrade from 85% efficiency to 90% in a breeze. We also know what else we have to work on to get those last few points in our reach for perfection."

Interestingly, four of the 25 staff members opted to leave, partially because of the exercise. More interestingly, the remaining 21 put another plan in motion which enabled them to absorb the four openings. The synergy system enabled every key player to have his and her say and each acted accordingly. Those with plus-plus values, attitudes, and behavior configurations were further satisfied. They were the majority, 21 of 25. The loss of four negatives helped the organization meld together and reach out for new opportunities in a critical aspect of medicine.

The climate for putting a new measurement practice into place is getting warmer daily. One of the biggest proponents is one of the biggest names in U.S. management—Harold Geneen. He's been hailed all over the world as a class business act. Recently retired, Geneen continues to hold the interest of many.

THE ESTABLISHMENT COUNTS, TOO

A "liberal" looking at the dais in the ballroom at the Waldorf Astoria in New York City this day would shake his head and say, *"Yep, that's Big Business...three-piece, blue suits with somber silk ties and very white, button-down, broadcloth shirts. These are the guys who know how to count."*

The "establishment" was there and the air fairly crinkled with excitement in anticipation of the featured speaker. Geneen, then chairman of International Telephone and Telegraph, was somewhat of an enigma but had the aura of an architect of civilizations and the certainty of a warrior general in battle. Geneen didn't make a lot of speeches and not surprisingly the Conference Board meeting was crowded with dark-suited aficionados waiting to hear what the executive's executive was going to say about business and its relationship to Government. When a young executive requested permission to record the address, Geneen said, *"Sure, just leave the recorder here, I'll turn it on when I get to the meat of it."*

Geneen usually got to the "meat" of things in a hurry. During his heyday, IT&T, which he jokingly referred to as International This and That, was the conglomerate that others envied, copied, and fawned over. And Geneen was the sole executor. His forte was to take a so-so company, give it his special management formula for success, and then literally watch it make the specific gains he set for it. The formula wasn't exactly a democratic form of business, but it worked for a long time under his guiding genius. While some executives dawdled over how and when to use the computer, Harold Geneen had it whirring at full speed.

The index, or evaluation of performance criteria, gave Geneen the power to control, with directness and certainty, a wide range of business activities that would have sent the best team of professional managers scurrying for cover.

When one of his 125 to 245 companies (the count varied with the year, as some came and some went) burped, Geneen knew about it. He usually asked that the Pepto Bismo be brought in with the diagnosis so little time would be wasted remedying the ailment. He maintained a visual accounting of each company and knew, in his head and on printout, what was going on at all times.

In his own retrospective of his career, recently published, he noted with some satisfaction that he rarely took an active role in the operations of the companies he oversaw. His role was to administrate the formula—the index of dollars and people and the relationship between them.

The sports world had long used index-like criteria to measure its heroes and heroines, for example baseball's famed "runs batted in" for hitters and "earned runs per inning" for pitchers, football's "yards per carry" for runners and "passes thrown/completed/intercepted" for quarterbacks, and so on for each sport. A "criteria" was slower to catch on in Big Business and Government (except for the military which historically has had a successful appraisal process).

Managing by index, a specific set of criteria which had meaning for each company in its industry, was a Geneen phenomenon, but it wasn't his exclusively nor did it apply only to big outfits like his. It seemed like his creation because of how effective he was at keeping track of his many and varied enterprises. He sure knew how to count. He made it popular in New York, London, Paris, and other money capitals. Maury Beschloss, on the other hand, made it work in Hammond, Indiana.

Maury Beschloss was not exactly in Harold Geneen's league—after all, he only ran one company—but he did a respectable job of it. The Hammond Valve Corporation produced $8 million a year selling specialty brass and other alloy valves. Beschloss worked in the dingy, industrial part of Indiana's Calumet Region where the orange colored sky came from Gary's open hearth furnaces, not from a lyricist's song book.

Those differences in atmosphere between Park Avenue and Front Street were really academic. They had one important thing in common—the sense to manage by the numbers.

Maybe Beschloss got his counting ability from athletics. He was sports editor of the Daily Illini as an undergraduate at the University of Illinois during the Butkus Era, and keeping track of the opposition's score was fairly easy—it was usually zero. More likely, Beschloss quickly learned numbers because he didn't have a lot of technical background in "values," so he figured out he'd better find some way to get a handle on keeping things under control. He came up with his own index.

THE VISUAL AIDS ARE IMMEDIATE

When you walked into Beschloss' office, the first striking note was how neat it was. It also was merey typical of what you'd expect for a president of a small, prosperous company. Nicely carpeted, smartly decorated, expensive but functional furniture and well-draped walls. Nothing elaborate. Until he began talking about the "index."

A touch of a button and the drapes parted, revealing a series of wall hangings of bar graphs, zig-zagging lines and pie charts. This profusion of visual colorings gave him an instant accounting of sales, production, rejects, overtime, safety, market shares and penetration, and other data significant to his way of measuring where the company was and where it was going. It was so colorful, even his face flushed, slightly, as he explained how it worked.

He stepped aside as an aide walked in and changed two charts as he continued talking. *"It's kept up to date, daily in some cases, weekly in others. Nothing goes more than two weeks. I want to know how many sales calls are made, where they're made, and how they went."*

"In the factory, I sit down with small groups of workers a couple of times a week and get their impressions of how things are going, as well as charting the numbers. We rotate the membership so each employee has a chance to talk over the course of the year," he explained.

Whether he knew it or not, Beschloss was developing his own synergistic system using the technical logic of numbers with the intuitive expression of how people felt about their productivity and job satisfaction. He was not waiting for trouble—he would anticipate it. He had limits and standards for each criterion so everyone who could influence the upward or downward markings on a chart knew how far they could go before expecting a call from Maury.

What Beschloss had discovered was that people performed better, himself included, if they knew the score. Less speculation occurred about projects, about where you stood in the scheme of things. People working at Hammond Valve had a healthy look about them. A bounce was in their step. Rarely did this situation come to fourth down, 20 to go on your own 10 with 10 seconds to play. Hammond Valve was a going concern that was not going to be caught napping.

What especially promoted this attitude was the fact that employees knew how the score was being kept, and they were given a lot of chances to input into the evaluation process. They knew the expectations and would work to them. It seemed like such a logical way to get work done. Geneen had fashioned the same concept into a practical format on a grander scale. Both, in their own stylistic way, made it work.

THE VISUALIZATION INDEX

What's in the index is not nearly as important as letting people know on what they are going to be evaluated. The index itself is no mystery. It can be as simple as Tommy Meehan's when, as mill manager for Crown Zellerbach Corporation in Camus, Washington, he drove to work each morning and exercised his index. On an early approach, he checked the smoke coming from the stacks. White meant something different than light gray, medium gray, or dark gray. (This, of course, was before air pollution control standards took this visual monitor away from him.)

Inside the gate, he noticed the tonnage on the loading docks, and after a few years could come within a whisker of the accurate count. As he turned toward his parking space, Tommy would survey the wood chip pile to see how inventory and waste were going. Before even parking the car, he was armed with relevant data to gauge the state of the mill, and could walk directly to the appropriate manager's office and inquire, *"What's being done about this?"*

Or the index can be as elaborate as IBM's, which compares each of its manufacturing installations, worldwide, on a set of ratios which promote high quality and quick delivery.

The index usually includes basic information such as sales, production, costs, and the like to determine unit and employee effectiveness. Or you can develop monitoring ratios that make sense for your particular business. Safeway Stores, Inc. uses a number of these: gross profit to sales, operating and administrative expenses to sales, and an even finer one to determine occupancy costs to sales. The successful companies, like IBM, use their own brand of ratios, including the strange one of secretaries to square feet of manufacturing area. Whatever works is the key. The more common ones are profit/equity capital, earnings to sales, sales/sales cost, employees/compensation costs, budget allocations/budget performance, sales/inventory, market/market share, plant capacity/plant utilized, etc.

They'll vary from industry to industry, and are sensitive to factors and features within them and as such make visual the multi-facets of the organizations. All these are critical to annual and longterm success. And they help people keep track of their performance in realistic ways.

VALUES AND SYNERGY CONNECTION

Any well-designed performance system helps weed out factors that have outlived their usefulness. By its nature, it concentrates energy and effort on the work being performed. It should not be used for any other purpose, although it can be a significant part of career pathing, management succession, and similar activities when thought through.

Today, appraisal of performance is often a negative and painful experience for both the appraiser and appraisee. This can be changed by using the core values as a base for the appraisal. Given this structure, the appraisal can be a positive, exciting and rewarding exchange.

In a society that has a penchant for counting every possible thing from MPG to RBIs to beans in a jar, our skill at keeping score on the professional at work is wanting. Our methods especially lacks precision when they come to measuring the intuitive side of people. They genuinely suffer in evaluating group performance, and in rewarding those in the group for their contributions.

On a societal level, evaluation is embryonic. For instance, what is the earmark of a good police department? Is it the crime statistics? Not really—those are generally more a product of the socio-economic pockets within the community. Is it number of arrests in relation to crimes committed? That's getting closer, but still not definitive enough. Is it a ratio of convictions over arrests? No, that's in the hands of the prosecution and the courts. Is it the number of patrol officers? Number of squad cars? Number of miles patrolled daily? What about prevention?

The fact of the matter is that the public doesn't really have good criteria to measure the effectiveness of its police. And the police don't either. They'll tell you that. This holds true for the postal service, welfare and social services, and any of the other entitlement programs paid for by federal, state, and local taxes. (A friend has often suggested that she could take the postal service, sell off the buildings and land it owns and use its other revenues to deliver the mail electronically to every television set in America while re-training its employees for productive work, and make money to boot. Tongue-in-cheek or not, you be the judge.)

The source holds true for most private sector businesses as well. Survey after survey points to the discomfort and dissatisfaction associated with boss-subordinate appraisal. The truth is that we don't have a good handle on the people side of doing business. Arthur Miller's *Death of a Salesman* toyed with the proposition and uncovered some realities that stand firm today—times change and you change with them, or get left behind.

The intuitive measures are very much in the same condition. We've been conditioned to leave intuitive development to chance, and Eric Berne's exceptional few rise to the top like cream in the bottle of unhomogenized milk. To avoid the isolation of being left behind or leaving to chance the opportunity of personal and group development, the core values, once understood, can trigger a shift in corporate life styles. Personal growth and organizational health can be connected and measured and are a basis for future action of humane and productive organizations.

INDEX FOR HEALTH AND PERFORMANCE

A health publication, *Prevention* magazine, which is widely respected and features how-to articles on health care for nearly three million readers, recently developed a *Prevention Index* for America. Publisher Bob Rodale commissioned Louis Harris & Associates to survey its readership to determine which factors were crucial to health and to develop a way to score people on their effectiveness in implementing these factors for themselves. The program also illustrated how much more could be done for better care—a potential index, if you will.

The *Prevention Index* proves to be an elegant starting place for a three-tiered evaluation format. By adding factors that the work group can track and aggregate cost factors for the corporation to be mindful of, a Health Care Index emerges. By taking it a step further, it can become a Health and Performance Index (Figure 11.1) that gives people more control over their working lives.

Let's follow the evolution. To become a system that overcomes the normal, single-dimensioned technical emphasis, it needs an equal amount of rational respect for job performance matched to an intuitive regard for personal health and vitality. Each alone would be a valuable contribution to corporate life style—together they provide a meaningful and visual tracking mechanism.

INDIVIDUAL FACTORS

A. Smoking

B. Blood pressure

C. Lipid levels (cholesterol)

D. Weight/Exercise

E. Vitamins/Minerals/Trace Element levels

F. Fat/Fiber intake

Figure 11.1. Health and performance index.

G. Salt/Sugar intake
H. Stress Factors
   1. Performance Skills/Project Results
   2. Alcohol/Drug abuse
   3. Absenteeism
   4. Sleep/Relaxation regimen
   5. Safety Record

WORK GROUP FACTORS

I. Cardiovascular incidences
J. Gastrointestinal incidences
K. Cancer
L. Hypertension
M. Mental health incidences
N. Substance abuses
O. Dental cases
P. Safety: Work/Home—Smoke detector, seat belt use, speed limit adherence, accidents, etc.
Q. Performance to Plan (H.1 composites; tallies the appraisals scores of all the exempt/professional employees)

CORPORATE FACTORS

R. Annual Premiums
S. Claims/Claims Paid (totals of I through P above)
T. Hospital Days per capita by operating unit (division, branch, department, et cetera)
U. Surgeries per capita by operating unit
V. Doctor Visits per capita by operating unit
W. Performance to Plan
   1. Profits/Revenues/Costs
   2. Market Share/Position
   3. Research & Development
   4. Corporate Citizenship
   5. Other

Figure 11.1. Continued.

The *Health and Performance Index* would, of course, be tailored to each organization, giving it a life of its own based on the realities and forces at work. Yet, some features are common to any organization, any work group and any person who works for a living. This combination of standard and unique factors is what gives everyone in the organization the chance to not only know what counts but how to count it. The Index enables each employee to see where his or her contribution fits into the whole. It is quickly and efficiently handled by the computer for timely reporting and can be accessed at any time for decision-making purposes. Senior managers can use unit-to-unit comparisons without invading personal privacy—a vital fact in that it helps focus on boss and subordinate confidentiality while providing masked statistics that can be decoded for practical use.

A NUCLEAR HOLOCAUST?

Psychologists and other students of human behavior credit a number of factors with feeding the current physical fitness explosion in this country. One factor that comes into play often is the realization that the world is susceptible to quick extinction from nuclear war and the individual's reaction, while somewhat naive, is to be as fit as possible while there is time.

Whether this subconscious drive is at the root of it or not, the reality is that more and more would-be crusaders are joining the personal survival race everyday. While some prefer to run alone or with pets, many find pleasure in working out with another fitness friend or even in groups.

The group phenomenon is worth examining. It may hold the key to some locked drawers in our cabinet of values. If we can figure out ways to better manage the group, we may discover answers to larger organizational issues.

For sake of argument, let's begin with the following three premises:

1. Unresolved personal conflicts cause distress, imbalance and less than effective use of intellectual, emotional physical and spiritual abilities.

2. Joining a group in this conflicted personal condition, an individual is apt to influence others in a less than positive manner (Values being plus plus, Attitudes being plus minus, behavior being plus minus) and heightens the chances for lowering productivity and job satisfaction for others. In other words, one bad apple can spoil the bushel and create conflict, i.e., distortion, distress, debilitation.

3. By alerting group members to these possibilities soon enough, precautions can be taken to avoid unnecessary conflicts and, in fact, efforts can be focused on issues, which abound, to direct energies toward goal and project completion, ala the Johns Hopkins experience.

If all the members of the work group (or family) understand this, are doing positive things for themselves, and are willing to assist in supporting each other's development, the stage is set for using the synergy system in its entirety—self-assessment, planning and, now, evaluation.

Peer evaluation has been around as long as dogs have chased cars and laid in the sun. It has undergone ridicule in some quarters, acceptance in others, and in the main continues informally as one, not the most, powerful molders of behavior known.

It can even shape up those with "bad attitudes," the Los Angeles Raiders being a case in point. Players like John Matuszak, Lyle Alzado, and others who couldn't "get along" on some clubs, fit in with the style and atmosphere created by owner Al Davis, who knows how groups work. At least, it looks like that from the outside. The team record as the winningest NFL franchise speaks for itself.

PATRIOTISM GENERATES ENERGY

An important concept to know is that taking a chance on some unknowns can pay off. Peter Ueberroth plied his systems magic at a more global level, dealing with a nation coming out of recession/depression mood in 1984. Time magazine credited his work with the 1984 Summer Olympic Games as the epitome of capturing a patriotic spirit caught in a web of world economic blahs and a feeling that America had become less than it once was.

Ueberroth set in motion a series of planned events that ignited the basic values of a nation. From the competencies of world class athletes, to the determined night-and-day running of the torch across village and towns and cities, to the teamwork of shuttling events around the maze known as Los Angeles, to commercial communications among the various sponsors and patrons, and the capstone of an unprecedented $215 million surplus, an economic first in Olympic history. The same man is the one who instituted the tough drug policy and practice in the national pastime.

The synergy resulting from connecting America's basic values did more to foster pride and patriotism than any event since the ending of WW II. The entrepreneurial Ueberroth, in studied humility, paid homage to the "plan." He had a game plan and nearly half of the world's population, 2.5 billion people, saw it carried out to near perfection—the litmus test of appraisal.

America stood tall, again. On, the 83 gold medals contributed to the shining moment. But for the first time in years, we could forget the Jimmy Carter "malaise" that gripped the land. We could close our eyes to gas shortages, hostage crises, and feel a national spirit that somehow had lost its way. Peter Ueberroth gave us a healthy taste of national synergy and renewed our faith in ourselves. The measurement of this success could be counted at several levels.

Not surprising Ueberroth, in his new role as baseball commissioner, is leading the fight against substance abuse. Once a crusader, always a crusader...a tall man in any league.

Less, however, is known about how peers can influence success, but some conclusions can be made. As in the situation at Johns Hopkins, a good group can very likely enable personal values development more quickly than can individual experience. Modeling and supportive action are a dynamic duo in this case. What you see is what you get. Starting or stopping smoking or drinking or drugs is a good example. Peer pressure can be good to help correct behavior, and it can be bad, as in a mob out of control. Planning, with appropriate input and discussion, then, keeps it on a fairly straight track that makes for accurate measurement.

Once the individual group members have started on their own development, have initial success, and convince themselves to take on larger issues, you've got the snowball coming downhill.

Some would say it's stretching things a bit to connect a need to an issue. Maybe so. When you put the synergy skills in the middle of it all, however, you begin to see an even clearer vision of what might be possible. Synergy is a two-step process that begins with a need, which develops into a skill through practice and can be applied cost-effectively to an issue at work or home.

Figure 11.2, contains three essentials in synergy—needs, skills and issues and illustrates the synergy process at work. Review the figure and look for the connections in your life.

NEEDS	SKILLS	ISSUES
Clarity	Job/Results Clarity	Role Clarity
Achievement	Work Plans/Schedules	Productivity
Industry	Problem Solving	Absenteeism
Integrity	Indicators/Standards	Quality
Control	Feedback/Evaluation	Costs, Overruns
Curiousity	Data Analysis	Creativity
Trust	Data Collection	Conflicts
Intimacy	Know Needs of Others	Labor Relations
Generativity	Close the Process	Management Succession
Self Identity	Know Self Needs	Stress, Substance Abuse
Autonomy	Keep Process Open	Leadership
Initiative	Risk Taking	White Collar Crime

Figure 11.2. Three essentials in synergy—needs, skills, and issues.

This is one way of looking at it. Take Self Identity, for example. The more you understand your motives, drives, and ambitions, the less you'll rely on drugs, alcohol, and other crutches. And the more you'll manage the stressful people and events in your life providing, of course, that you're also developing the eleven other needs, skills, and issues.

Initiative, which cultivates your risk taking skill, will be enhanced when you take on troubles such as White Collar Crime, Employee Rights, and other sensitive but high-cost issues in work units. Of course, connecting two skills, such as Self Identity and Initiative, will bring about more energy for the necessary change.

That's for openers. The next step is to work up a project out of each, then track the progress with a system of core values as explained earlier.

EVALUATION IS A MATTER OF FEEDBACK

Two factors are crucial to any synergistic appraisal process. Since all messages between two individuals come with a content or overt form and a process or covert form, the measurement format must include both. For instance, when you tell the cop who just stopped you for speeding that you're on your way to a fire, he can accept the social, content, and overt part of that message, and let you go. Or he can read the psychological, process, covert side, which tells him you're lying, and give you a ticket.

It's the same when you tell your boss that "extenuating" circumstances prevented you from having the report completed on time. He can accept the face value, left brain, rational explanation, or he can challenge it on his previous experience with your being late, check it with his/her right brain intuition, and give you a pink slip.

Or, in the case where the boss believed you because of a previously established confidence, you would get into a dialogue about when the report will be ready, like in 30 minutes.

So you see that scoring depends not only on the core values but also on a scale of relevance. Earlier you saw how all relationships develop from the Status Quo through Questioning to Awakening to Confidence and, finally, to Synergy, a five step climb. Score it on a 5-point Likert scale—two lows, a middle and two highs—and each value can be reflected in the output from your work effort.

Using the previous example, if you had a Status Quo or Step 1 relationship with the boss, you might be in deep trouble. Likewise, if you had reached Confidence or Level 4, you'd be able to work out something quickly that would maintain the relationship and accomplish the project. By knowing the intimacies of the relationship, you are in a better place to get the work done and improve the relationship at the same time. Without that knowledge, you're likely to lose on both ends. Let's look at a classic situation.

Nancy B. wondered why Mark, her supervisor, suddenly seemed so distant. She had worked for Mark at Systems Protection Services (SPS) in Atlanta, Georgia, for nearly four years and gradually had built a strong relationship which he dubbed a "great double-play combination." Building the relationship had not been easy. Nancy was quiet and not taken to speaking up and Mark found it hard to open up at first, too. He had not wanted to be "boss" but was promoted to supervise a group of technical specialists as the company grew rapidly. He certainly did not want to manage females, whose place he felt was other than in high tech systems security, a complex and sometimes risky profession.

Mark graded each employee's performance according to the firm's formula and Nancy soon came out on top after some early problems communicating with Mark. They worked it out as Nancy learned that Mark liked to hear all or most of what took place with a client after installation of one of the systems began. So they spent considerable time together even though eleven others also were installing systems. Mark liked how Nancy could give a factual accounting, as well as her sensitivity to how things impressed her at another level. Before long Mark began to rely on her more and more, and the tougher clients soon became her specialty.

The mutual respect grew as Nancy appreciated Mark's hints and clues of what she could do to advance herself in the company. He hated to lose her, but knew she had the stuff to take his job and SPS was opening regional offices across the country—quality supervisors were at a premium.

She was, he thought, a diamond in the rough and could probably move up a couple of notches in the rapidly expanding SPS hierarchy.

Besides taking at least one night school class a semester, Nancy followed Mark's advice and read several publications, including *The International Journal of Security & Investigation*, and followed closely the research of the Assets Protection Institute and other professional organizations in their industry. For fun, she took a pottery class and got into "throwing." She felt her growth as a person and as a professional in a thriving and exciting field. She was, however, perplexed at Mark's behavior.

Maybe it was drugs, she thought. Marijuana and cocaine were rampant in the industry, and while she had experimented a couple of years ago, she decided not to go along with the crowd. She wasn't sure where Mark was on the issue. She only knew that their relationship at work had fallen off. She didn't like it, and even though it took a lot of effort, she decided to confront him.

They had lunch in a nice restaurant, sat in a quiet, out of the way booth, and she reviewed the relationship. Nancy did not push or corner Mark, but she did express her feelings. He rejected the premise at first and said nothing was wrong. But he knew her ability at sizing up situations at both levels and, when she offered to help, to stand by him whatever was up, he admitted to having a serious problem.

It was drugs. Only he had gone a step further. Embezzlement. He was stealing from a client to pay for his soaring drug habit. He sobbed out the details, one by one. Nancy stayed calm and listened. Mark felt relief oozing out of his body and mind as he confessed his sins. Nancy gave brief but cogent counsel. Mark listened, agreed, and they walked out together to seek professional help. (*The Wall Street Journal*, 2/7/85, had a similar story on Page 1.)

The issue of white collar crime is a growing one, experts numbering it as the third-largest dollar volume item in the country after war-related expenditures and illicit drug traffic. And the growing concern is that drugs and white collar crime are closely connected.

The cost to business and government, for crimes like Mark committed, is somewhere between $55 and $110 billion, depending on the source.

Nancy had stumbled onto it with Mark and he had a problem to iron out, which he did, and after restitution, got off with probation and a ruined career.

The situation could have been different if a vehicle had been operative to prevent Mark's impulse from swaying his otherwise sound judgment. Nancy could have acted sooner, too, if she had been watching with her intuitive side. With her usual concern and Mark's usual reliability, yes things could have been different.

GETTING CLOSER, SOONER

Nancy and others could have used the visual aid shown in Figure 11.3 in sorting out the perceived troubles they were having. This simplified scoring version of **The Values Survey** introduced in Chapter 9 is called **Values Tracking,** Figure 11.3.

PROJECT NUMBER & DESCRIPTION		
	Rational	Intuitive
Competence	————	————
Determination	————	————
Teamwork	————	————
Communications	————	————
Economics	————	————
TOTAL	————	————

SUMMARY:

Figure 11.3. Values Tracking System.

The ***Values Survey*** provides you with a satisfaction/frustration level based on current events in your life. The survey results serve as an index for either work or social aspects of one's life. By using the ***Values Tracking System*** as a measurement index for any project, it becomes a workable tool that can provide focus and eventual achievement.

While both the rational and intuitive aspects of each value are graded on each project, the total gives both the gradee and grader an instant understanding of how well the work is going and equally importantly, how well the individual is getting along with others involved in the project.

The summary allows space for dramatic contributions such as cost and health data, or any issue you identify from Figure 11.2, Column 3. (Scores are referenced 1 to 5—the Likert scale—five being high, and correlated to the Stages of Relationships model described in Chapter 6 and Figure 6.1.)

By tying this project performance scoring system to the health and performance index mentioned earlier, changing corporate life styles becomes a reality for those standing tall at work and home.

SUMMARY

Those who know the appraisal process control their own destiny.

One of the most thoughtful, criteria-based evaluation systems is when health and performance indices are tied together, using values as the base.

The index is incomplete without both content and process measurement criteria of all the jobs and functions of the organization. Values, which are linked to skills which allow for task completion, can be the basis for appropriate employee appraisal, organizing a sense of how the family is doing.

By grounding the organization in its own values, the people become more a part of the process and willing to contribute as much as their potential allows them. Scoring makes the contributions more tangible and easier to reward. Growth becomes secured in this environment.

CHAPTER **12**

STAR SPANGLED SPIRIT

The father's waiting room was almost empty as Walt Ward fiddled with a cigarette, anticipating news from the delivery room. What started out to be a great day had turned into a living nightmare. **"Can't they get anything right,"** he hissed through his teeth.

It had been 12 hours since he left the alternative birthing center, where the plan was to have the baby naturally, using the modern LaMaze method. A miscalculation and miscommunication between doctor and nurse forced abandonment of a good idea. Next, they induced labor and took Ellen to the delivery room to use forceps in the delivery.

Walt was allowed to watch part of that procedure, but when it failed, he was advised to go to the waiting area. After that setback, the doctor said the baby would have to be taken in a caesarian section. **"That probably means no more babies for Ellen,"** Walt reckoned.

Walt had smuggled a bottle of champagne into the waiting room. He sloshed another pouring of champagne into the paper cup and stared darkly at the bubbling liquid. **"This was gonna be a memorable day,"** he thought. **"All I want now is Ellen and the kid to be okay."**

As he sat, waiting, he felt the hate and anger building in him. The more he drank, the easier it came. **"The system is sick. This hospital, these doctors, the process is plastic. God, what went wrong? What did I do wrong?"** He felt cheated and spent and with that he threw the paper cup at the window. It made a quiet, dull "plop."

Later, Walt looked down at the dark-haired creature sleeping quietly in the crib. Tears filled his eyes. **"My son,"** he blubbered. Mother and child were fine.

As the ordeal began to melt from one part of his mind, he knew it would never leave his memory. Walt was too much of a realist and too pragmatic, though, to be stymied. He reached for a pen and began drafting a life plan on the back of an envelope for Thomas William Ward, his son.

A CRUSADER'S PERSONAL GAME PLAN

Riding the wave can be fun for the accomplished surfer, a little dangerous for the inept and exciting for the onlooker. It's a matter of being skilled, knowing the conditions, feeling confident and going with the flow—letting go of excess baggage. For the crusader, the same thing occurs when dealing with the ups and downs of emotional and spiritual issues—the crux of life on this earth.

Life is a total package and each aspect needs to be planned. Overcoming fears, guilts, and anxieties are the issues to manage. We do so by generating the creative energies we once commanded in our innocence of youth. The plan leads to accomplishment. Nothing is taken for granted, including the excitement and the outcome.

Yet, everybody's had those days when getting into stride seems impossible, the button falls off a coat, the check that's in the mail doesn't arrive, the dog gets sick on the carpet just before the guests arrive, or the boss decides to send you to Newark on your daughter's recital day. Planning: Wouldn't it be nice if everyone had the same inclination to work toward greater harmony?

Balance may be a relatively new business and life style phenomenon, except maybe for accountants who live on balanced credit/debit and other statements or the dancer who relies on tip of the toes walking for style and grace. While it's true that our pioneering forebears also took a turn on the balance wheel to settle this country, much of recent history tells us about our imbalances—the deficit, civil rights, haves and have nots, and other social disparities such as booze and drugs—remain.

On a more remote but equally distinctive parallel is the discipline exercised by the Indian and Oriental warriors centuries ago, long before the pioneers began to settle the West. Chogyam Trungpa, the Tibetan Buddhist, described the Shambhala process in his book, *The Sacred Path of the Warrior*. We can paraphrase the master and learn from it—another connection from history to the present—a way of standing tall.

A WORKING MODEL

Four basic "dignities" or conditions embody the Shambhala warrior: Meek, Perky, Outrageous and Inscrutable—one building on the previous one. The words, however, need more description because they don't fit the American idiom.

Meek, for instance, is seen in the warrior as simplicity, an uncomplicated and completely approachable self. Meek also means self-contained without arrogance, inquisitive without bias, and relaxed yet alert. The Meek are conceptual, see the total picture and will complete the task no matter what because of these characteristics.

The assertion is that Meek walks like the tiger of the jungle, easily with eyes softly focused, listening to the sounds of the environment, Graceful, not stalking.

Compare that description with the synergy skills of data collection, data analysis, and knowing the needs of others. Then add the core value of determination to the description. You'll see a possible connection. Curiosity, trust, and intimacy are the traits being developed along with the concept of wisdom and serenity. Once mastered, these skills and this motivation for quality brings the apprentice into the warrior's camp.

Once on the grounds, the trainee moves toward **Perky:** on energetic, ongoing discipline, a youthful and enjoyable status. It is seen in an uplifted self, artful in action, rather than being timid and fearful of the future and the unknown. A Perky person takes delight in reality—the here and now—rather than shrinking from it, knows the appropriate standards for situations, harbors no self doubt, and is in balance with rationality and intuition. He or she has no fear of survival, walks like the snow lion with an assurance of direction, and suffers no paranoia.

Couple Perky with Meek and you see a warrior who is gaining in confidence, is comfortable with life's contradictions and ambiguity, and is growing in respect of order and spontaneity. You also can imagine a warrior standing tall—the aims are similar, if not the same. A warrior stands tall among peers.

Compare Perky with the synergy skills of knowing self needs, indicators and standards, and work plans and schedules, and the value of competence. The warrior/crusader is advancing toward his or her potential through achievement, integrity, self-identity, and a growing integration of human and technical skills necessary for total living in a complex and changing world.

Outrageous is a condition that builds on the first two. it goes beyond the duality of hope and fear; it allows freedom to risk, to change the process, and to talk directly and honestly to others, providing them with needed straight talk. When one goes beyond hope, the emotional roller coaster ride ends. Hope brings either euphoria or despair. The Outrageous warrior/crusader needs neither.

An Outrageous person, then, does not wait for hope or fear, sees obstacles as opportunities, negatives as a challenge, which brings a tremendous relaxation. No anxiety, only horizon exits. Mr. or Ms. Outrageous stops to lend a hand to others with patience and encouragement.

Compare Outrageous to the synergy skills of risk taking, closing the process, evaluation, feedback, and the value of communications. A warrior/crusader can encourage freedom through initiative, generativity, control, and open dialogue.

The last dignity of the warrior/crusader is **Inscrutability**. This does not mean a blank wall or deviousness, as many Americans might suspect. It means being noncommittal with a sense of humor, playful when solving problems. An Inscrutable person is never depressed, because the possessor of this dignity exudes opportunity for all concerned. No preconceptions here. Just standing tall.

The Inscrutable person is clear, open to the world, fearless and takes one step at a time. This warrior/crusader knows what to do even if others don't, so teaching others while moving in the right direction is part of being Inscrutable. He or she knows when to let go and is not afraid of failure because the next step brings the right path in sight. Like the dragon, the Inscrutable one is patient and calm until the energy is needed to right a wrong.

Compare Inscrutable with the synergy skills of clarity, problem solving, keeping the process open and the value of teamwork. You'll notice that a warrior/crusader at this level keeps expectations in order, solves problems without intense reaction, and is autonomous while being a part of the group effort. The synergistic outcome is the value of economics—the profit from learning the crusading warrior's way.

The four dignities can be developed in today's crusader by training in and acceptance of the twelve skills and the five core values. Anyone willing to be productive and a healthy person can use this model. It means dropping all the gimmicks and tricks one has learned to offset being authentic. As in the Stages in Relationships, you move forward at your own rate of development, until you are at Synergy—the crusader's perch. . . tall among the trees.

ESTABLISH A BASELINE

In the days when the annual physical examination was reserved for senior executives and thought to be a key man "perk," the corporation operated on an industrial relations model developed in the 1930s. Today, this antiquated model is being replaced in thoughtful organizations with the "smorgasbord" approach to benefits, giving single parents, dual career couples, and traditional families what coverage is most sensible for their specific situation. The dual emphasis is on prevention—an essential for changing your life style—as well as treatment.

Prevention of disease is an advocacy for health. This approach will have stress-reducing influence, because the cost-conscious employer knows that Ben Franklin spoke well when he talked about penny wise, pound foolish. Restricting check-ups only adds to long-term medical costs, as well as undermining personal development. Check-ups are for everyone.

As mentioned earlier, the exam need not be the high-tech, high-cost diagnostic, but an old fashioned, comprehensive, hands-on poking around to see what's what. The fancy stuff has its place in selective cases where a serious problem is suspected. Otherwise, the general practitioner approach can be most efficient to catch a problem or one that might be. GPs and mobile multi-phasic health testing offer excellent service meeting the most stringent of medical codes. And the price is affordable for large groups, especially those which have people in satellite locations.

Once the baseline health information has been established, then a program such as the Health and Performance Index (see Chapter 11, Figure 11.1) can be cost effective and productive. Any ongoing organization development system which includes coordinated and equal emphasis on both health care and on-the-job performance will be useful to keep employees fit and satisfied.

A number of awareness tools are around to help senior managers create a systems approach for their specific situation. The key is to create interest and action through self-assessment and evaluation. When people have input to the plan and the evaluation follows accordingly, the results are stunning.

Exams and self-assessments need not be limited to just the physical. Peak performers who want to maximize their abilities and continue the search for their potential also will test their emotions and mental and spiritual prowess.

These exams are keyed on the status of personal balance. A lopsided wagon wheel may have been funny in old Western flicks, but not so in day-to-day living. Medical and organizational behavior authorities agree that physical, emotional, intellectual, and spiritual balance is essential for good health and peak performance wherever you live and work.

If you have a body that is genetically designed to live those idealized 120 years, you'll need to exercise common sense as well as exercising your body. Moderation, and listening to experts as well as your own body talking, will help. Whether you've momentarily lost your purpose and seek new directions or are in more serious need of repair, the check-up and self assessments are the starting line.

An interesting conclusion reached by medical authorities here and abroad, especially the British Medical Association, is that the high-tech, computerized affair is not the popular answer. The best solution is the old-fashioned hands-on exam to look at the condition of your brain, the blood vessels, and the heart. All can be done without a lab test or x-ray.

Without a single lab test, a doctor can diagnose hypertension, diabetes, heart ailments, hardening of the arteries, bleeding tendencies and more. For instance:

- By listening to the heart, the doctor hears the four valves at work and can determine their efficiency.

- By looking into your eye, a check of the optic nerve provides early detection of many brain diseases.

- By looking at the blood vessels running down the optic nerve, it's possible to see arteries and veins and determine high blood pressure damage, diabetes, and bleeding tendencies.

- By listening to the chest, the doctor evaluates the noises, fluids in the lung and, if murmurs, whether serious or not.

- Rectal exam discloses 15% of bowel cancers as well as allowing a check-up on a man's prostate.

- An abdominal check gives status on the liver, spleen, bowels, and related lower intestinal health.

Massive high-tech testing can, and does, turn up problems that don't exist. Healthy people often have abnormal results in one test or another because normal generally means a range in which 95% of the population, by age group, falls. You may be in the 5% outside one set of limits without being in trouble. This will be determined by further examination or tests by the doctor—all probably essential, on one hand, but extremely costly on the other.

Too often, the choice is to take more expensive tests which prove that you are one of the special, healthy people who happen to fall into a 5% category. If the doctor feels strongly that you require additional tests and lab work, so be it.

Evidence is abounding that four critical test groups are essential and do not require costly lab work. They are

1. cervical cancer,

2. hypertension,

3. bowel cancer, and

4. breast cancer.

For healthy people, these four can be detected by safe simple, and accurate tests, the ultimate criteria. Early detection usually proves beneficial for useful treatment. In some instances, say for lung cancer or emphysema, no treatment is known and some testing may be more harmful than good. Some troubles of the past, such as tuberculosis, which required harmful x-ray testing, have subsided and hardly anyone recommends testing for them. If your doctor suspects something more serious based on preliminary examination, it's best to go along with his experience and judgment. The safe, simple, and accurate rule is a sound one to follow as long as you feel in the pink.

Being informed of your biological status is essential as one lesson to keep away from substance that can harm you.

THE NEXT STEP IS MENTAL HEALTH

Mental health is most commonly linked to insane asylums, kooks, and retardation. These, unfortunately, are popular misconceptions. Mental health is a combination of intellectual and emotional soundness. For your game plan to have maximum clarity, you can determine soundness, in part, through the values and synergy surveys within this book. These surveys will give you a preliminary status report on your stress levels and satisfaction/dissatisfaction ratio.

Less than 3% of the national population qualifies as certifiably insane, a small but painful figure. The remaining 97% may have ups and down when it comes to emotional problems, but these are controllable and not socially crippling. Usually they are rectifiable and can be treated professionally. Most of these maladies can be prevented by paying attention to behavior patterns, and many, if not all, are stress-related. And **distress precedes substance abuse in most cases.**

As pointed out by Dr. Friedman's and others' research, **intensity** is a major factor in appropriate behavior. What you have discovered about your intensity from the **Synergy Skill Survey** (Chapter 9) provides you with adaptation options. By being aware of which of your skills are being used to the extreme, you can begin to reduce excessive effort with the intention of bringing less distress into your life, just like a warrior would.

A word of warning: now that you know appropriate behavior can be considered within the 15 to 25 intensity range, you may try to appear balanced without adapting the feelings that drive the behavior. In other words, you must understand your values first and connect them to attitudes which will then prompt new behavior. Adapting behavior alone will not last for any length of time and may get you into more trouble than you now experience.

For example, if you were prone to let off steam when frustrated, got to be known as a "hot head" and suddenly began curbing this natural outlet without getting at the cause of the frustration, this new behavior might lead to a different set of circumstances, equally as unrewarding. You need a system to care for yourself which works at your values, attitudes, and behavior simultaneously.

Even doctors, who know better than most what harm can be brought to the body through abuse, continue to have troubles with addiction. Those who are the ones who generally have mental and emotional disabilities. On the other hand, those who are totally healthy are exhibiting a crusading spirit.

CRUSADING SPIRIT . . . Standing Tall in a Crowd

Elisha Gray II came from a long line of board chairmen, or so the story goes. His great-grandfather invented a telephone and was a few minutes behind Alexander Graham Bell in filing for a patent. Undaunted, the great-grandfather started an electrical supply company called Graybar which still produces a nifty income today. Another Gray headed up the Corning Glass Works in New York and so it came as no surprise that Elisha (Bud) Gray would eventually find his own bright place.

Bud started with Sears and Roebuck after college, but soon figured out that Big might translate as Slow, even for one as gifted as he. Whirlpool Corporation supplied Sears with washing machines and other appliances and it had the qualities that appealed to young Mr. Gray. He moved from Chicago to Benton Harbor, a trip of less than an hour by car but eons when measured in industrial significance in those days. Bud Gray would do a lot of traveling while leaving his mark.

The appliance business in America in the 1950s was a hodge-podge of giants like General Electric, General Motors et al., and small fry like Tappan, Servel, Norge, and others. Whirlpool, which supplied nearly two-thirds of its output to Sears, was nearer the giants but lacked an identity of its own . . . until Bud Gray got cooking.

The record shows that the company grew from less than $700 million in annual sales in the early 60s to better that $2 billion in the early 70s under Gray's winsome leadership. How did he do it? Those who were there at the time know the answer. He let people have their way. His favored expression in those exciting and action-filled days was, *"If we can make one of six or seven ventures pan out, we can compete with anybody."* His "ventures" always included new teams being formed to handle a project. He liked the idea of putting together different players with new roles to create excitement and results. His success ratio proved that synergy does and can exist in large bureaucratic situations on a large scale. His key can be yours: trust yourself first, then trust others.

Any game plan must be shared with others who can give you feedback and thus help keep you on track, especially during the early stages when you need encouragement. Forty-Niner Coach Bill Walsh spends a lot of time developing his game plan and is generally credited with being the offensive planning genius of his time. The Inscrutable Walsh shares his genius with the team and when all other factors are equal, the Niners win. Without a way to share the plan, it would be a wasted effort.

So the same is true with successful CEOs like Gray, Geneen, Beschloss et al, who challenge and support their chief lieutenants in carrying out the strategic plan. They talk turkey, straight ahead language, even the forgotten visual language. They walk like lions and tigers and can be dragons. This approach leads to changing the way of bureaucracies.

INTEGRATING SKILLS AND MOTIVATION

Too many business operations seem to be run under a shroud. The veil may be enticing in some fashions, but not in the world of work where clarity is key. One department head won't share views with another for fear he or she will "get ahead" in some secret competitive race for favors.

In certain family-run operations, where you'd expect that behavior to be least likely, brothers and sisters take sides against each other with the expected outcome of poor performance and demise. "Boy, I showed them." That's a throwback to infantile days. It also forces lower level executives and employees to take sides which, by its very nature, is divisive.

Clarity is the first developmental skill because without it all the rest are destined for sporadic success. Ask a good hitter what's most critical in getting on base and the answer overwhelmingly is "keeping your eye on the ball." If you don't know where the ball is you aren't going to hit. It's as simple as that. It's the first and cardinal skill in most sports and at work.

Clarity can be boiled down to expectations. What do you expect from the time and energy you put in at work? Realistically. What does your supervisor expect? What does your spouse want? Your children? Don't guess or assume. Ask in a dialogue over time. He or she may not have thought it through either and may need time to figure it out. Don't give up after one try.

At another level, the boss's boss may have a different set of expectations for you and your boss. Find out. Encourage that dialogue as well. See if all these fit into the corporate life style. If yes, you're on your way. If not, do something constructive about it. Failing that, update your resume.

This little Conflict Resolution Model (Figure 12.1) tells a lot about expectations and conflict resolution.

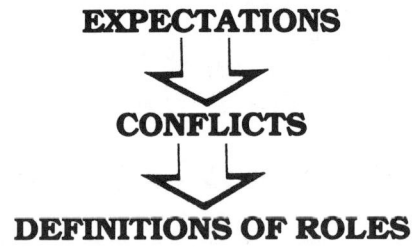

Figure 12.1. Conflict resolution model.

Unstated or unclear expectations will invariably lead to conflicts between individuals and groups. If you and your son or daughter are only assuming a curfew hour and the kid comes strolling in at midnight when you thought it was a ten o'clock night, a conflict will follow.

Conflicts at home and work are as common today as a cold in winter and just about as easy to resolve. For the cold, you take two aspirin, get some rest, and call the doctor in the morning if complications result.

For a conflict, it takes a more rigorous strategy and often with the same results . . . it goes away with some careful attention but not simply with the passage of time. Conflicts are either confronted head-on or with third party assistance to reach resolution. Left alone, conflicts fester and cause serious **disease** in family and organizational life. As a warrior/crusader would, resolve the conflict without anxiety, intensity, and emotional bias.

A virtually fool-proof way to rid a specific conflict from your life is to have both parties involved sit down and look at what is going on and gain agreement of what each must do to turn the negative into a positive flow of energy. By determining each one's role for reaching common ground, the conflict can generally be turned around, or at least you can gain agreement to disagree.

The most common conflict, however, goes on within the individual—the inner conflict associated with tentativeness.

MEASURED COMMITMENT

Activity

By doing the activities that follow, get a feel for game plan format. Don't do any writing or doodling at this time, but merely assess what has to be done.

Think about the changes you'd like to make in your life style, or the adjustments in how you are living. By putting your thoughts on the brain's "back burner" you're allowing for incubation, that essential step for creativity, as Einstein noted.

Once this is in place, get into soft focus. You can accomplish this by a series of simple techniques:

- Give yourself at least 30 minutes preparation time.

- Do a few stretching exercises to limber up.

- Do two or three minutes of deep breathing with a slow release.

- Once your mind has quieted and your body and mind are better connected, pick up a pencil and turn to the synergy worksheets.

Do as the ancient warrior crusader would and work on the aspects of yourself that follow Trungpa's ideology—data collection, data analysis, and needs of others, along with the value of determination. Working one at a time, spend two minutes writing a stream of consciousness, and then three minutes on a preliminary draft. Do these in pencil, as you will enhance them later. At your next session, do three more, as indicated earlier, or use your own perceptions of which should go first, second, and third. Work at this until you have completed initial drafts for the entire 12 and the five values.

The preliminary strategic plan will be the base you need to turn these into a tactical action plan when you meet with your peer group and, later, you will have a substantial plan to present to your supervisor—your part of changing corporate lifestyle.

Writing in pencil also helps to keep the process open a while longer while you collect information on where to practice the skills development, and as feedback is given on how well you are doing.

The important element is to work in short, specified time frames, while in soft focus, to develop your peak performance patterns. As your performance improves, the pattern becomes reinforced by your own observations of how well you are doing as well as by the feed back you'll be receiving from those around you. These may not occur immediately, so keep the process open for at least three weeks. Dr. Maxwell Maltz, in his book "Psycho-Cybernetics," gave credence to the idea that it generally takes 21 days to trade off a bad habit for a good one. When all other things are considered, however, recent research reveals it takes three years to be assured that it is ingrained yet susceptible to subtle influences necessary to keep it attuned. The same can be said for the crusading life style.

USE SHORT TIME FRAMES

Although no specified time outs are in a work situation, as occurs in sports, you can call "time" when things are not on track. For instance, most projects run into deadline trouble because not enough time is given to the planning of the project. The boss may want something done in two weeks that, in reality, is a three, four, or six week research effort, or possible longer.

As you learn to do more in shorter time frames on segments of a project, you still may need to realize that Murphy may have been right in telling us that ". . . it's gonna take longer than you planned" for the total effort. Murphy's Law being what it is can be useful if we use it rather than merely laugh at its consistency and our own inconsistency.

Time is a clock to many, while to more serious planners time is a way of knowing how to proportion the specifications of a project. By using time frames in a plan, you're more likely to produce the result you want.

INCLUDE CALCULATED RISK

Maslow pointed out that people move up a stair step of hierarchical needs as they progress in self development. when basic biological needs of air, water, food, and so forth have been met, we move to safety and security, then to belonging and love, then to self esteem, and finally to what he called Self Actualization, doing what we are best suited to do.

What he didn't have time to say was that when we reached the fifth level, we move into a new territory, so to speak, and find ourselves at the bottom step of a higher order of needs. The comfort of success suddenly leaves us as we start all over again.

That's why a calculated risk is essential. Most of us resist change because it's discomforting. Some stay in the comfort, feeling incapable of another trek into the unknown. The growth cycle, unfortunately, must be paid for with a little pain. To make it as painless as possible calls for a reduction of risk, a rational sorting through the options.

Rehearsal is the best way for a professional to reduce those unintended bloopers. Just as professional athletes work diligently before each game, so the business, technical and artistic professionals need to practice to fulfill their potential.

CONNECT TO OTHER SYSTEMS

As you perceive yourself more as a system today, you will be able to latch onto other systems in your organization to benefit yourself, them, and the whole. Without that understanding, your action would be a charade, something less than reality.

Four systems to include in your crusader's game plan are

1. a support group,

2. a mentor,

3. the organizational supervisor, and

4. the core/project cluster.

The core cluster is the work you're being paid to perform. Part of it can be structured into projects while some of it, the core, cannot. Do as much of it in projects as you can and the remainder will be core work, usually. In rare cases, the core will remain larger than project transformations, but only rarely.

A writer, for instance, has a core of research, development, writing, editing, and submission of a manuscript. He or she counts the number of projects—books, articles, short stories, et cetera—that are intended for publication. The core of each project remains the same, while the projects can differ greatly.

Knowing that core work and projects are the base of your personal system, then you can think of how to connect to other systems where you work. Develop these connections according to the sphere of influence—a visual reminder that you manage your time and energy to stay in balance and get the return on energy investment that will keep you as stress and drug-free as possible.

Once you've made the connections that will transmit critical information for your career, it's time to look one more time at professional skill development.

REALIZING YOUR POTENTIAL

Even with the best of intentions, skills development can get lost in daily routines. What makes sense, then, is to have routines established that enhance the developmental process, just like the routine you go through every morning on awakening.

While rubbing the sleep from her eyes with one hand, a friend walks to the bureau, find the sweat socks and jogging suit, and sits down to pull them on. After putting on the running shoes, she finds her way to the kitchen for a quick glass of juice and powdered protein. Then out the back door, across the yard, and out to the street for a five-mile jaunt. About a quarter-mile into it, she clears her mind and gets in touch with how her body is doing. The routine is going well and she starts to enjoy it.

This friend doesn't spend a lot of energy thinking through the first ten minutes of this routine. It has become habit. No chance for sidetracking here. Pure routine helps her to get into an enjoyable place each morning. It gives her the clarity she needs to begin each day fresh and to get on with her job of building winners. She's a willing supervisor—a crusader.

You can do the same for each of the skills if you want to assure yourself positive routines that won't require a lot of energy to get started, and to maintain good habits. By looking at each skill from a different perspective, you'll add substance to your crusader status.

The following twelve examples—six under rational skills and six under intuitive skills—are food for thought.

Rational Skills

1. Job/Results Clarity. Pete Rose was making $800,000 a year for making outs seven of ten times at bat. We pay someone $35,000, $45,000 or even $75,000 and expect performance of seven, eight, nine, or even ten of ten. Is that a realistic expectation? Detail your three-year plan and talk it over with your boss and mentor, and develop realistic expectations. From these talks you'll gain the clarity necessary for the long run.

Like the jogging supervisor, you'll need to do something every day to keep these expectations from getting clouded or distorted. It may be a physical caring for your body, or it can be an intellectual review of the plan or an emotional rigging of one or two projects to refresh your motivation.

Whatever you choose, it's usually best practiced alone. At least until you gain some confidence it it. Clarity lends itself to solo flight...a soaring into clear skies.

2. Work Plans and Schedules. A play opening on Broadway usually plays New Haven or Hartford first after weeks of rigorous rehearsal. Professionals in most other disciplines recognize the value of practice making perfect, or near perfection.

Only in management and working with people does rehearsal seem out of character and genuinely resisted by the players. Once the plan is written, it tends to be buried in the stack of Things To Do Today.

The game plan demands daily practice on each facet. Each meeting is a chance to practice specific strengths, yours and those of others in the meeting. Going to strength keeps the process alive and fresh, rather than fretting about What-Might-Have-Been. When you schedule a conference with one other person or a group, define the strengths to be used by all those involved and you'll soon see shorter meetings, increased satisfaction, and more output.

When you have clarity about outcomes based on individual needs, you'll meet deadlines without the usual anxieties. Your calendar will highlight your schedule of relaxation, exercise, and quiet time. The theory is that if you write it down it will likely get done.

3. Problem Solving. Wehrner Von Braun, records show, suggested 67,500 changes in the V-2 rockets he was building during WW II before he was even partially satisfied they would work to perfection. His way of debugging a new system called for a lot of problem solving before the fact. We spend millions each year in re-calls, re-work, rejects, and law suits rather than preliminary problem solving.

Problem solving the American way is exciting and gives inveterate problem solvers a chance to stand out. But at what cost? Problem solving, as you know, is based on Industry . . . knowing how things work. By being a preeminent problem solver, which means taking time to research effectiveness, you will gain a reputation for cost-effectiveness that will be more durable than the fire-fighting variety.

Use problems to teach your skills to others less experienced. You can coach the beginner to do both before-hand and after-the-fact approaches to this skill, connecting Autonomy and Industry for another systems approach to Synergy.

4. Indicators and Standards. Gemologists have a sensible way to assay gold, give diamonds a fancy rating, and otherwise denote the quality of stones, gems, and jewels. They have built the system over time and it's accepted throughout the world. Again, in the world of work we have trouble developing a standard system for sizing up the quality of Management on both left and right brain criteria.

Most of the standards are based on left brain interpretation of values and skills, especially economics and problem solving.

In world class track and field, all the standards are there to be broken—twenty feet in the pole vault, eight feet in the high jump, and so forth. The standards for running a business will vary according to the business but very little when it comes to the people side. All individuals and work groups require special care and treatment but it doesn't vary by industry.

People will beat the "standard" given the opportunity to sharpen their skills and enough time to practice and test themselves. The current standards, the skills to be sharpened, time, and support all become the system to set new standards. Use your current skill standards as hurdles to be topped in your daily run for the smell of roses.

5. Feedback And Evaluation. Like the Laws of Nature, people and work seem immutable. The selection process insures that only the fittest will survive. This message is conveyed swiftly over and over again.

Yet we fail to use the fundamental and recognized tools available to improve our selection process. If Drucker and others are correct in saying that only people, of all the resources of the organization, can grow, where is the state-of-the-art in feedback and evaluation, which are two primary cultivators of human resources? The *Health and Performance Index* (See Chapter 11) seems to be the one.

Make a contract with several people you know who can be crucial to your work performance. Exchange feedback and evaluation on the evolution of your work projects. Don't worry too much about the final evaluation. Your boss will undoubtedly carry most of the weight on that aspect. Concentrate on the process of how you are each performing. If you're off 5 degrees, correct the course and don't take it personally.

6. Data Analysis. The whirring of computer disks is the sound of the close of this century and probably of the beginning of the next. Data can be crunched at mind-boggling speed, reports chunked out of printers with monotonous regularity and accuracy. Still, some people wear green eye shades and sleeve garters, ignoring what can be learned from past successes and failures.

While the best time to sit down and review game film is as soon after as possible, many organizations don't even take snap shots, let alone critique what took place. Somewhere on the calendar of events, a time and place to figure out what went right and wrong must be inked in. It's not a blaming discussion, but a calm period for learning from recent, accountable history.

Intuitive Skills

7. Data Collection. A former colleague was told never to take off his coat when visiting a superior's office. He never did. He never got beyond the formality in relationships, either. People tended to make fun of this Stuffed Shirt, and he never became the "superior" that he wanted so much to be.

Whether the relationship is formal or informal, the idea is to establish trust. This doesn't come about by whispering a magic phrase or sharing a fraternal hand grip. It comes from moving up that pragmatic stair step of listening, questioning, deciding, working on and gaining the confidence that leads to trust. Trust in yourself is the starting place. The more trust you have, the more you can share and expect in return. Keeping promises to yourself is a good trust exercise. Meeting work plans and schedules are other good trust experiences.

8. Knowing Needs Of Others. On a football recruiting trip to the Southwest, a young assistant coach tempted a prize athlete with a variety of proven inducements. None worked. The young halfback with size and 4.4 speed would not commit to a letter of intent. He later enrolled at a smaller college where he had been asked several seemingly insignificant questions about his needs by a young but wiser assistant coach.

The best way to get people on your side is to give them what they need. The best way to find out is to ask them. Sometimes they may not know, so you'll have to watch them for a while and then suggest some things. Or maybe you have to ask the same thing in a different set of ways before it strikes a chord with them. Don't give up. Keep researching the issue. It's vital to your success.

9. Close The Process. The pressure to succeed is so strong in some companies that competition becomes internecine. One place overcomes this by regularly swapping team members. Loyalty stays with the organization, not with one manager. Decisions are made so that everyone wins. people tend to grow faster in the climate. It fulfills the concept of Generativity, which calls for leaving the place better than you found it.

Not many places promote teams over individuals yet, but the day may come. Until then, you'll find it advantageous to remind yourself that decisions made for short-term results can return to haunt you next year or the year after. Thinking in collective terms, such as the product or service, the people making and buying, and economic returns, will produce more quality decisions.

10. Know Self Needs. A researcher visiting a Mid-western mental hospital recently found most patients there to be either totally certain of who they were or totally confused. Only a few fell in between. Those who were sure often were deluding themselves.

Those who were confused frequently were unable to stop long enough to take a good, clear, and hard look. The researcher figured that this applies, on a smaller scale, to most of us. Being absolutely certain of who you are may result in cutting out your chance to grow to full length.

No one knows his or her potential. It's there to be developed through risk and testing. You'll add to your data base and increase understanding. To find out where you want to go, what you really want out of life, and how to get it takes a systemic approach. First you look and see what you value and then you look at what's most important. Then prepare yourself, with help from others, to battle for your fair share.

11. Keep The Process Open. The chaos normally associated with the creative process causes tradition-bound people to shudder. They don't "see" the order and are in dismay when creators attempt to explain it. Creative types, however, exhibit great discipline to achieve results. They'll try this and that, tossing out and throwing in. In the end, it's a balance that wins out. True learning comes when we have discipline arising from initial chaos. A system is in all that blind fury.

A lot of stress is caused by deadlines that are unrealistically set, much like standards that are arbitrarily established. The time to exercise autonomy is up front. Ask for, then demand that time frames consistent with what's practical be set. Murphy was right in saying it always takes longer than you planned.

Work, though, is best accomplished in short time frames. Projects with a known start, middle, and end usually hit on target. Without this orientation, work takes longer, adds to stress, and increases costs on several levels. Do yourself a favor. Borrow time for planning and you won't be strung out trying to keep the wolves at bay.

12. Risk Taking. Two young people walked along a swollen creek. One suddenly stopped and asked the other to jump in and swim across. *"Can't swim,"* came the honest answer *"Even if I could, I wouldn't." "Scared, huh?"* the other surmised. *"No. I'm already on the side I want to be on,"* the young sage said.

Knowing which side to be on is assessing risk in an adult manner. Pushing the process too hard can cause dire consequences, like jumping in over your head. Moving the process to a point where you want it to be is calculating the risks.

Taking little risks can condition you for larger moves. Like talking to a stranger. Making a new friend, intentionally. Learn how to swim, speak Spanish or take a vacation to a place you've never seen. Go ahead with a project on a hunch after thinking through all known options. Standing pat can sometimes be the most risky. Unless, of course, you've been dealt a straight flush.

A nice family get-together could be attendance at a drug and alcohol clinic given by your local school or police department. Everyone could learn the biological and pharmacological harm that can be cone by substance abuse and could serve as good discussion starter for all family members.

WHAT'S EXPECTED OF ONE WHO STANDS TALL

So the proceeding are some guidelines for one who stands TALL—a crusader's personal game plan—a systems approach to professional and organization synergy. Whether you are left brain dominant, intuitive, or, by some wonderful set of circumstances, find yourself in harmony with others in the world around you, try to be more of the architect that resides in you somewhere . . . waiting to spring out and educate and entertain others. You don't need a guru to become whole.

CELEBRATE

Whether you decide to go this trip alone or will embark with a crew of co-workers or family, plan to celebrate some of the outcomes. A friend I know spends an evening with the sunset over San Francisco Bay as many as 50 times a year . . . each a reward to herself for a job well done. Another associate pours himself a favorite potion of non-alcoholic beverage to quench a thirst. Another takes the dog for a run on a trail.

Whatever you choose to do, think about it. What pleasant experience will fulfill your desires after making progress on the plan?

Maybe you can trade-off smoking for good health, put the money saved into a celebration fund, and award it to a favorite charity after a year. Maybe the entire group could contribute and share in the economics of it in some way. And remember you'll want to update it next year this time.

SUMMARY

The personal game plan is a way to gain more control over your life and to enjoy more moments of it with those around you.

Start with a total assessment of yourself. Use the data from the surveys to draft your plan.

The plan is most likely to succeed if you share it with others and involve them in your achievements.

By knowing your values and skills, especially the intensity associated with them which can cause distress, you have a power to change some of the elements of life that now disturb you.

Celebrate the fact that you were a fundamental part in altering the corporate and personal life style in a positive and profound way—a way of standing tall.

INDEX

A

Accident
  recovery 108-9
Achievements 76
Acquired Immune Defiency Syndrome (AIDS) 15
Adams, J. 172
Addiction 4-6
  alcohol 4
  cost 8
  "hard stuff" 4
  smoking 4-5
Addicts
  new lifestyle 106
  putting life together 100-4
Adler, A. 66
Adolescence
  paradox 14-5
Adults
  learners 83-5
  teachers 83-5
Agenda
  hidden 108
Aids
  visual 282-3
AlaNon 50
Alcoholics Anonymous (AA) 7, 23, 50
Alden, W.F. 20
Aldrich, V. 108-9
Alpha 32
Alzado, L. 289
Amino acids 252
Anderson, W.W. 38-9
Anti-Drug Abuse Act 21
Approach
  systems 193-4
Art
  of inclusion 152-4
Ashanti Tribe 262-3

Ashe, A. 174
Autonomy 12, 13, 78
Awareness 106-8, 111

B

Balance
  reaching a state of 89-90
Bangham D. 102-4
Bangham J. 102-4
Baseline 301-5
Beckoning 33
Behavior 13, 72-3
  Type A 171-2, 176, 232, 243
Bennett, W.C. 271-2
Berne, E. 98, 137, 157, 175-8
Bertken, T. 67
Beschloss, M. 281-2
Bias, L. 15-6
Brain
  left 198, 200
Buscher, F. 69-71, 73

C

California Youth Authority (CYA) 96
Carbohydrates 252
Career
  dual 121
Carlson, D. 161
Carter, J. 290
Case
  Jardine, J. 36-8
  Jardine, S. 40-4
  Ward, T. 3-4,35-6, 63, 93-4, 119, 145-6, 163-4, 175-6, 181, 207, 261-2
Castenda, C. 110
Cayce, E. 29

Celebrate 320
Cellulose 252
Change
    interconnection to learning 69-70
Characteristics
    concentration 147
    skills 147
Choices 58-61
Christ 104-5
Clarity 76
Close the process
    interpretations 225-6
Coast Guard 21
Cocaine 16
    hotline 18-9
"Coke" 16
Commitment 205-321
    measured 309-11
Communications 66-7, 202
    definition 237
    interpretation of scores 239-40
Competence 66-7, 202
    definition 236
    interpretation of scores 238
Competition 193
Comprehensive Crime Bill 21
Computer
    era 195-8
Concentration
    power of 171-2
    relationship 172-4
Conference Board 200
Conflict
    managing 168-70
Conflict resolution
    skills 164-5
Conflict Resolution Model
    Figure 308
Conover, R.E. 47
Control 76
Coping 244
Core value
    definitions 236-7
Core Value Profile, *Figure* 269
Core Values
    interpretation of scores 238-40
Core/project cluster 312
Costs 18, 20, 56
    addiction 8
    health care 183-5

Crack 16
Creativity
    discipline 79-80
Crimes
    drug-related 96-102
Crockett, B. 268
Crusade 30-3
Crusader 33
    definition 39-40
Curiosity 77
Cycles 57, 58
    nature's 48-50
    nine-year 49-50
    personal 48-50

D

DARE, project 21
Data analysis 317
    interpretations 223
Data collection 317
    interpretations 224
Davis, A. 289
Decision 113
Decision-making process 61
Dedication 141
Degnan, B. 97, 98, 99-101, 109, 125
Delta 9 THC 16
Determination 66-7, 202
    definition 237
    interpretation of scores 238-9
Development
    physical 251
Dewey, J. 29
Discipline
    creativity 79-80
Divorce
    member 120
Dowling, M. 147-52
Drucker, P.F. 195
Drug Enforcement Administration (DEA) 16
Drug testing procedures 26
Drugs 9

E

Economics 66-7, 202
    addiction 17-21
    definition 237

Edison, T. 107
Education
   ongoing 68
Ehrhard, W. 66
Einstein, A. 79
El Paso de Robles School 96
Elkin, D. 241-5
Ellington, D. 90-1
Ellington, E.K. 90
Ellis, D. 100-1
Employee
   appraisals 277
Encounters 250
Energy
   accessing 154-8
   patriotism generates 289-92
   source of 154
   spiritual 110
   works through personality, *Figure* 72
Entrepreneurs Alliance 66
Erickson, E. 10-3, 74, 79-80, 92, 128-31, 132
Evaluation 277, 292-5, 302, 316
   performance criteria 280
Evidence
   statistical 4-7
Example
   See Case
Excellence
   search for 12-4
Expectations 13
   standing tall 320
Expression of self 12

F

Factors
   corporate, *Figure* 287
   individual, *Figure* 286-7
Families
   different types 134-6
Family
   balance 137
   caring 136-8
   corporate involvement 122-3
   divorce 120
   dual career 121
   head of household 121
   responsibility 138-9
   television 139-40
   single parent rate 120-1
   status as a unit 122
   troubles 138
Farnham, M. 157
Fats 252
Fear 57
Feedback 292-5, 316
Feedback/evaluation
   interpretations 222-3
Ferguson, M. 29
Fiber 252
Focus
   hard 174
   soft 174
Fonda, J. 28
Ford, H. 29
Freud, S. 65, 66
Friedman M. 28, 171, 232, 305
Fromm, E. 57, 58-9, 94, 196
Fulbright Fellowship 65
Fulbright, W. 64-5

G

Game Plan
   crusader's personal 298-9
   parents 133-4
Game playing
   If It Weren't for You 157
Game "2/4/2" 142-3
Geiselman, T. 40-1
Geneen, H. 279-83
Generativity 77
Gephart, R. 55
Gettman, J.B. 28
Giles, B. 53-5
Glasser, W. 100
Gold, M. 18-9
Goldwater, B. 55
Graphs
   three thermometer, *Figures* 214, 215
   synergy skills, *Figures* 212, 213
Gray, E. 306-7
Greeks 168
Green, V. 99
Groder, M. 98, 101
Guidelines
   values 131-3

Index 325

H

Hall, M. 42
Harrison, T. 99
Hart, G. 140
Head of Household 121
Health care 190
    cost 107
    practice 106-8
Health and Performance Index 286-8, 296, 302, 316
Health Maintenance Organizations (HMOs) 53
Herrmann, N. 81, 267
High
    natural 95
Hirschman, A.O. 81
Hofer, E. 68, 146
Holliday, B. 74

I

Impatience 12
Inclusion
    art of 152-4
Index 280-1
    health 286-8
    performance, *Figure* 286-7
    visualization 283-4
Indicators 315-6
Indicators/standards
    interpretations 221-2
Indulgence
    self 155-6
Industry 11, 76
Influence 80-3
    sphere of, *Figure* 80
Initiative 78
Injury
    recovery 108-9
Inscrutability 301
Integration 190
Integrity 76
Intensity 305
Intensity score
    Synergy Skills Survey 229-32, *Figure* 230
Intimacy 77

Investing
    in children 266
Irving, J. 89
Issues
    Figure 291
Ivory, J. 49

J

James Logan High School 264, 267
Jane 255
Japanese 107, 113
Jardine, J. 36-8, 42-4, 49, 51
Jardine, N. 40, 42, 51, 55
Jardine, S. 40-4, 42-3, 49-51, 54
Jean 255
Job/results clarity 314
    interpretations 218-9
John S. 253-4, 257
Journal
    keeping 154
Joyce, J. 141
Jung, C. 66

K

Keegan, J. 25
Keyes, R. 89
King, M.L., Jr. 95
Knowles, M. 84, 87

L

Latham, R. 124-31
Law enforcement
    teaching 166-8
Learners 83-5
Learning
    experiential 85-6
    interconnection to change 69-70
Lerman, L. 266
Lifestyle
    community 188
    corporate 188-90, 199-201
    corporate model, *Figure* 202
Link
    missing 191
Lippitt, G. 152

Listening to
    harmonics of life 270-1
    message 269-70
Litt, B. 152-4
Los Osos Cottage 96-101
Love 46-8
Lowe, G. 97
LSD 20, 70

M

MacLaine, S. 270, 273
Maltz, M. 71, 73, 311
Management
    business unit planning 197
    lesson 197-8
    matrix 197
    objectives 197
    self 208-9
    strategic planning 197
Marijuana 16, 18
Maslow, A. 68, 75
Matuszak, J. 289
McCain, J. 55
Measurement
    universal 278-9
Meek 299
Men
    against women 86-7
Mental health 305-6
Mentor 189-90, 245-6, 312
    guidelines 245
    mentoring 245
Message
    listening to 269-70
    non-verbal 108
Mind
    changing 201-4
Minerals 252
Model
    parent-child discussion, *Figure* 169
    personality, *Figure 248*
    serenity 158-60
    values/skills/issues, Figure 202
    wisdom 158-60
Moon, W.L.H. 90
Motivation
    integrating 307-9
    nature of 65-8
    values 187
Moynihan, D. 120
Mucins 252

N

National Organization for the Reform of Marijuana Laws (NORML) 16-17
National Press Club 64
Nature's cycles 48-50
Navajo Indian 129
Needs
    Figure 291
Needs of others
    interpretations 225
    knowing 317-8
Negatives
    overcoming 246-7
    turned into positives 147-52
Neoteny 144, 189
    definition 140
    model for family growth 140-2
Neurosis 60
No
    not enough 35-62
NORML 28
Nuclear Holocaust 288-9
Numerology 49
    instructions 52
Nye, D. 166-8, 169

O

O'Laughlin, J. 264-5
Oils 252
Openness 140-1
Options 106-8, 112-3
    growth 117-204
Outrageous 300-1

P

Paradox
    adolescence 14-5
Parents 104
    game plan 133-4
    responsibility 138-40
Participation
    art of disciplined 264-5
Path
    synergistic 205-321
    to power 104-5

Patience 141
Pattern
    systemic 112
PCP 20
Peak
    performance 229-32
Peale, N.V. 29
Pectin 252
Performance
    appraisal 284
    index, *Figure* 286-7
    peak 229-32
Perky 300
Perot, H.R. 138
Personality
    energy, *Figure* 72
Peter, Paul, and Mary 95
Pfaff, G. 83
Plan
    strategic 192-4
    tactical 192-4
Planning
    business unit 197
    process, introduction 262-4
    strategic 197
Poem 101-2
Potential
    realizing 313-20
Power
    path to 104-5
Preferred Provider Organizations (PPOs) 53
Pressure
    reacting to 156
Prevention 24-5, 302
Pribram, K. 82
Price, K. 156
Problem solving 315
    interpretations 220-1
Process
    alpha 106-8, 111-2
    close 318
    events 165
    introducing the planning 262-4
    keep open 319
    stretching 275-96
Process open
    interpretations 227-8
Professionalism 190
Program
    nutritional 252-3
Promises 113
Pygmalion Concept 167

Q

Questioning
    stage of relationship 149

R

Reality
    treatment of the thrill 96-7
Relationship
    concentration 172-4
    interpretation for four stages 240-1
    scores on four stages 236
    stages 148-52, *Figure* 148
    stress 172-4
Religions 46-7
Repass, J. 185
Responsibility
    parents 138-40
Rhythm 233
Risk 89-90
    calculated 312
    taking 319-20
Risk taking
    calculated 189
    interpretation 228-9
Ritual 112
Robbins, T. 140
Rockwell International 22
Rogers, D. 15-6
Rosen, R. 56-7

S

Schedules 314-5
Schools
    change 271-3
Self
    getting to know 232-3
Self identity 78
Self image 214
    Figures 214 & 215
Self needs
    interpretations 226-7
    know 318
Self-assessment 302-3
Self-identity 12

Self-image
    interpretations 216
Serenity 158, 160
Sesame Street 145-62
Shambhala
    process 299-301
Sheehy, G. 49
Shulberg, B. 65
Sidetracker 254-8
Signs
    of the times 163-80
Skills 74-9
    conflict resolution 164-5
    Figure 291
    integrating 307-9
    interpretations for effectiveness 224-9
    interpretations for efficiency 218-29
    intuitive 317-20, *Figures* 75 & 230
    learning observation 170
    rational 314-7, *Figures* 75 & 230
    twelve 301
Snyergy skills
    graph, *Figures* 212 & 213
Sphere of influence
    Figure 80
Sphere of Influence Cone, *Figure* 256
Spirit
    kindred 119-44
Spirit
    star spangled 297-321
Stage
    alpha 106-8, 111-2
Stage of relationship 301
    awakening 150
    confidence 150-1
    model 296
    synergy 151-2
Standards 315-6
Star
    shine 208-9
Stathis, G. 49
Status 89
Status Quo
    stage of relationship 148-9
Stock, R. 44-6
Stress 192, 244
    relationship 172-4

Stress management 131
Struggles
    inner 155
Stuart, J. 99
Students Against Drunk Driving (SADD) 25
Style
    interpretation for professional 217
    professional 215, *Figures* 214 & 215
Substance abuse
    economics 115
    supply 115-6
Supervisor
    organizational 312
Support group 312
Synanon Game 99
Synergy
    needs to create 251-3
    needs, skills, and issues, *Figure* 291
    profile 215, *Figures* 214 & 215
    values connections 284-5
Synergy connection 284-5
Synergy Profile 233
    Deborah, *Figure* 243
    interpretation for 217
Synergy Skills Survey 209-229, 305, *Figure* 210-1
    intensity score 229-32, *Figure* 230
    scoring interpretations 216-29
    summary, *Figure* 210-11
Synergy 82, 92, 124, 199-200, 290, 301,
Systems
    approach 193-4, 199-200
    approach, definition 200
    bureaucratic 201-4
    connect to other 312-3
    support 189

T

Talk
    straight 254-8
Talker
    incessent 156

Index 329

Teachers 83-5
    television 146-7
Teaching
    law enforcement 166-8
Teamwork 66-7
    definition 237
    interpretation of scores 239
Teamwork/family 202
Television
    teacher 146-7
Threat
    external 182
Three Thermomether Graphs 214-5
Time 174-5
    frames 311
    structure 175-9
    use of 179
Toffler, A. 208-9
Tough Love 22
Transactional Analysis (TA) 99
Transactional Analysis Seminars 98
Transitions 190
Triggers
    changing 247-51
    emotional 249-50
Trungpa, C. 299
Trust 10, 77

U

U.S. Department of Commerce 53
Ueberroth, P. 289-90

V

Values
    core 202, 301
    guidelines 131-3
    motivation 187
    survey 295-6
    synergy connection 284-5
    tracking, *Figure* 295

    tracking system 296
    work 188
Values Profile 233-41
Values Survey 233-41
    core values 236-40
    interpretation 237
    scoring 236-40, *Figure* 234-5
Victim
    association 157-8
Vinovich, J. 99
Visualization
    path to power 155
Vitamins 252
Von Braun, W. 315

W

Ward, T. 3-4, 35-6, 63, 93-4, 119, 145-6, 163-4, 181, 207, 261-2, 275-6
Ward, W. 297-8
Water 251
Wisdom 157-9
    definition 158
    serenity 158
Woodyard, S. 90
    collaborative 276
Work plans 314-5
Work plans/schedules
    interpretations 219-20
Worlds
    collision of 182-3

Z

Zones
    distressive and depressive 231
    overactive and suppressive 231
    productive 231-2

ABOUT THE AUTHOR

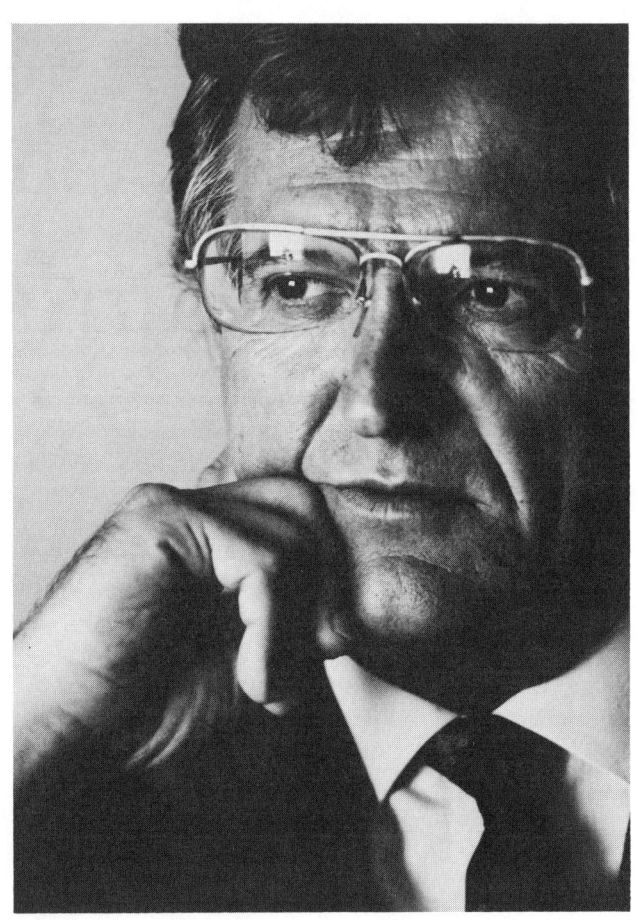

ROBERT T. WALL

ABOUT THE AUTHOR

Robert T. Wall is a native of Chicago and developed basic values growing up and working in the Midwest before moving to California in the mid 1970s.

His career covers investigative and news reporting at the *Decatur Daily Democrat* and *The Fort Wayne Journal-Gazette* both in Indiana; corporate and press relations at Wheelabrator-Frye Corporation in Mishawaka and at Public Service Indiana in Plainfield; organization and management development at Whirlpool Corporation in Benton Harbor, MI, and Crown Zellerbach in San Francisco, CA, and a consulting career with more than 100 clients including IBM, Shell Oil, the Port of Oakland, Fred S. James Company, the U.S. Air Force, the Bank of America, and others.

Wall served on faculties at Indiana University, Golden Gate University and Antioch Graduate School of Education besides being the first director of GGU's Institute of Productivity Improvement, where he also was the youngest member of the Board of Trustees.

The father of four, Wall lives in the East Bay of San Francisco and is working on his first novel.